Sciatica
and
Chymopapain

Sciatica
and
Chymopapain

John A. McCulloch, M.D., F.R.C.S. (C)

Former Assistant Professor
Department of Surgery
University of Toronto
Attending Staff
Division of Orthopaedics
St. Michaels Hospital
Toronto, Ontario, Canada
Assistant Professor
Northeastern Ohio Universities
College of Medicine
Akron, Ohio

Ian Macnab, M.B., Ch.B., F.R.C.S. (Eng.), F.R.C.S. (C)

Professor
Department of Surgery
University of Toronto
and Chief
Division of Orthopaedic Surgery
The Wellesley Hospital
Toronto, Ontario, Canada

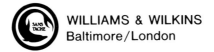

WILLIAMS & WILKINS
Baltimore/London

Copyright © 1983
Williams & Wilkins
428 East Preston Street
Baltimore, MD 21202, U.S.A.

Made in the United States of America

Library of Congress Cataloging in Publication Data

McCulloch, John A.
  Sciatica and chymopapain.

  Bibliography: p.
  Includes index.
  1. Intervertebral disk—Hernia—Chemotherapy.
2. Chymopapain—Therapeutic use. 3. Sciatica—Chemotherapy. 4. Injections, Intradiscal. I. Macnab, Ian. II. Title.
RD771.I6M36 1983   617'.56061   83-10482
ISBN 0-683-05754-5

Composed and printed at the
Waverly Press, Inc.
Mt. Royal and Guilford Aves.
Baltimore, MD 21202, U.S.A.

Preface

Low back pain is a symptom; sciatica is a symptom. A herniated nucleus pulposus may cause either symptom. Either symptom may be caused by a host of other diseases (Table 7.1). Every day of our professional lives many of us have to wrestle with these symptoms and their causes. Not infrequently, in spite of the best clinical and investigative efforts the diagnosis eludes us. This is the thread of frustration common to any practice oriented towards spinal pain. It is hoped that the first half of this monograph will add something to your understanding of sciatica as a symptom and a herniated nucleus pulposus as a cause. It is in this group of patients that chymopapain has its greatest benefit.

Back pain is second only to the common cold as a cause of time lost from work (1). It has been estimated that every workman loses about 4 hours per year because of back pain. Each year 300,000 operations for low back pain are carried out on the North American continent at an average estimated hospital cost of $5,000.00 per patient and professional cost of $1,500.00 per patient. When one totals lost time costs and medical costs, low back pain is a multi-billion dollar industry. Competing for attention and seeking influence in this cause are many types of professionals and nonprofessionals, including medical doctors, osteopaths, chiropractors, acupuncturists, naturopaths, massage therapists, and even fortune tellers.

The supposed beneficiary of these efforts, the patient, stands bewildered, a victim of controversy within the professions and conflict between the disciplines. All the patient wants is freedom from low back pain so he can return to a desired lifestyle. Sometimes the patient gets less, when an ill advised, ill conceived surgical procedure fails to improve, or aggravates, his symptoms. As a result an aura of fear and hesitation towards back surgery has built up over the years, and when the patient is presented with the prospect of surgery, he may seek other avenues of treatment. The patient then enters the world of the unknown, where available to him are all manners of treatment.

One such treatment, which for many reasons has occupied the world of unknown medical care, has been chemonucleolysis. In 1964, Lyman Smith (2) suggested that enzymatic dissolution of the nucleus pulposus by the intradiscal injection of chymopapain could overcome pressure on a nerve root produced by a ruptured disc. Discolysis, or as Smith suggested, chemonucleolysis, a nonsurgical method of removing offending disc material, was born.

Very rapidly arguments regarding the safety of this technique and its efficacy changed chemonucleolysis into a cause rather than a technique of treatment. Surgeons took sides on philosophical rather than on scientific grounds. Widely divergent views were expressed. Some considered

v

the technique to be a very valuable addition to our therapeutic armamen-
tarium, whereas at the other end of the spectrum some surgeons stated
that chemonucleolysis was not only useless, but it was downright dangerous. During this time, the mere mention of the term, "chemonucleolysis," could rapidly change friends to acquaintances. These diverging
views, rigidly held and hotly contested, were almost invariably based on
impressions only.

The second half of this monograph is to assist in the resolution of the
chymopapain controversy. It is based on the authors' combined experience with 7000 patients who have undergone discolysis with chymopapain
over a 14-year period.

While the authors have remained convinced of the efficacy of the
procedure throughout this time, opinions and support for the procedure
have followed a roller coaster ride with many setbacks in acceptance by
scientists, surgeons, health industry regulators, and patients. The low
point occurred in 1975 when the United States Food and Drug Administration, faced with unfavorable double blind results of a chymopapain
trial (3), prevailed on Baxter-Travenol to withdraw their New Drug
Application. With this unofficial stamp of disapproval, discolysis with
chymopapain quickly fell from favor, especially in the neurosurgical
community.

The comeback trail for chymopapain has been long and hard but new
evidence arising out of better controlled studies is now emerging in
support of chymopapain (4, 5). Discolysis appears to be here to stay as
an alternative to surgery. In fact it is the first of a number of percutaneous
spinal surgical procedures that will be appearing in the future.

The art of surgery is to make the correct diagnosis which will form the
basis for invasive therapeutic efforts on your part. Although it may seem
remarkable in this age of sophisticated medical technology, on close
analysis, the greatest problem with chemonucleolysis has been the inability to make that sometimes elusive correct diagnosis of the underlying
pathology. The reasons for this are the basis of the first part of this
monograph.

Chemonucleolysis is only of value in overcoming sciatica due to compression of a nerve root produced by a prolapsed intervertebral disc. If
the leg pain is only a manifestation of referred pain from segmental
instability, then chemonucleolysis will be of no value whatsoever. If the
leg pain is indeed radicular in origin but is due to apophysial stenosis or
bony root entrapment, then dissolution of the nucleus pulposus by the
intradiscal injection of chymopapain cannot be expected to overcome the
patient's symptoms.

Chemonucleolysis is of no value whatsoever in the treatment of degenerative disc disease with referred sciatica pain not associated with root
compression. Peripheral vascular disease may produce a leg pain that on
occasion may mimic sciatic root compression. This syndrome obviously
cannot be overcome by chemonucleolysis.

There are no words in the English language that describe pain. The patient can only describe the disability the pain causes. Disability caused by pain is closely related to the patient's emotional content. In some patients, the emotional content of the disability is of paramount importance. In better emotional health, such patients would not be disabled by the pain they experience. In this group of patients, any treatment, by surgery or by chemonucleolysis, *directed solely at the disease process* is unlikely to rid the patient of his bothersome burden of pain.

This, then, is the purpose of the book. It is hoped to remind readers of the clinical picture presented by a patient with a ruptured intervertebral disc giving rise to nerve root compromise and, having done this, to establish criteria for treatment by injection. At the same time, contraindications for the use of chemonucleolysis will be described in detail. The technique of the intradiscal injection of chymopapain will be described and the immediate postinjection management of the patient discussed. Finally, the results of chemonucleolysis in this center will be recorded to enable the clinician to give some form of informed prognosis to his patients.

This book has been written with unmitigated dogmatism. When a new technique is started, in order to establish its value, rigid criteria must be set down and followed. Otherwise, it remains as a philosophical concept rather than developing into a reliable technique with readily reproducible results.

It has been said that the only hero, in heroic surgery, is the patient. The authors would like to acknowledge their indebtedness to the first group of patients who allowed themselves to be treated by a technique that they knew was still in the stage of investigation (6). We also thank the Department of Photography and Art at St. Michael's Hospital; Mary Hogan, research assistant; Char Cary, for hidden talents; the nurses of the operating room, recovery room, and the outpatients who participated in this study. Thanks are also due Ms. Sara Finnegan and Ms. Barbara Tansill for their light-handed editorial help without which these typewritten pages would never have been transformed into a monograph which we sincerely hope will take the "black magic" out of chemonucleolysis and make it into an easily understood scientific approach to the treatment of sciatica.

Finally, we would like to thank Williams & Wilkins for giving us permission to reproduce many of the diagrams (Figs. 1.1 to 1.11, 5.1, 5.2A, 5.6 to 5.12, 5.14, 5.21, 6.3, 6.5, 6.8, 6.9, 6.13, 6.15, 6.17) from the monograph, *Backache,* published by them in 1977.

JOHN A. MCCULLOCH
IAN MACNAB
Toronto

References

1. Kelsey J, White A: Epidemiology and impact of low back pain. *Spine* 5:133, 1980.
2. Smith L: Enzyme dissolution of the nucleus pulposus in humans. *JAMA* 187:137, 1964.

3. Schwetshenau PR, Ramirez A, Johnston J, *et al.*: Double-blind evaluation of intradiscal chymopapain for herniated lumbar discs. *J Neurosurg* 45:622, 1976.
4. Fraser R: Chymopapain for the treatment of intervertebral disc prolapse—a double-blind study. Presented at the International Society for the Study of the Lumbar Spine, Toronto, June 1982.
5. Smith Laboratories, Inc. New Drug Application 18-663. Submitted to the United States Food and Drug Administration, March 10, 1982.
6. Weiner DS, Macnab I: The use of chymopapain in degenerative disc disease: A preliminary report. *Can Med Assoc J* 102:1252, 1970.

Contents

		Preface	*v*
CHAPTER	1	Anatomy	1
CHAPTER	2	Epidemiological Aspects of a Herniated Nucleus Pulposus	12
CHAPTER	3	Biological Basis of a Herniated Nucleus Pulposus	15
CHAPTER	4	Biomechanical Concepts in Herniated Nucleus Pulposus	18
CHAPTER	5	The Pathogenesis of Sciatica	24
CHAPTER	6	The Clinical Syndrome of Lumbar Root Compression Due to Disc Rupture	54
CHAPTER	7	Pain and Disability	82
CHAPTER	8	Chymopapain—Chemistry and Tissue Reaction	97
CHAPTER	9	Selection of Patients for Chemonucleolysis	103
CHAPTER	10	Technique of Chemonucleolysis	128
CHAPTER	11	Post-Chemonucleolysis Course	182
CHAPTER	12	Adverse Reactions to Chymopapain	196
		Epilogue	208
Appendix I		Patient Preadministration and Discharge Instructions for Chymopapain Injection	214
		Index	219

CHAPTER 1

Anatomy

It is a convention observed by most authors of medical texts to start the book with a chapter devoted to the anatomy and embryology of the subject covered. In many instances this is a form of Brownian movement having very little purposeful significance.

The purpose of this introductory chapter is to remind the readers of anatomical terminology and to correlate the gross anatomical features of the lumbar vertebrae to pathological changes of clinical significance. We have chosen to modify the usual format markedly and have assiduously avoided detailed description of morphology.

We can consider each vertebra as having three functional components: the vertebral bodies, designed to bear weight; the neural arches, designed to protect the neural elements; and the bony processes (spinous and transverse) designed as outriggers to increase the efficiency of muscle action.

The vertebral bodies are connected together by the intervertebral discs and the neural arches are joined by the zygapophysial joints (Fig. 1.1).

The discal surface of an adult vertebral body demonstrates on its periphery a ring of cortical bone. This ring, the epiphysial ring, acts as a growth zone in the young and in the adult as an anchoring ring for the attachment of the fibers of the annulus. The hyaline cartilage plate lies within the confines of this ring (Fig. 1.2).

The intervertebral discs are complicated structures, both anatomically and physiologically. Anatomically they are constructed in a manner similar to a car tire with a fibrous outer casing, the annulus, containing a gelatinous inner tube, the nucleus pulposus. The fibers of the annulus can be divided into three main groups: the outermost fibers attaching between the vertebral bodies and the undersurface of the epiphysial ring, the middle fibers passing from the epiphysial ring on one vertebral body below, and the innermost fibers passing from one cartilage plate to the other. The anterior fibers are strengthened by the powerful anterior longitudinal ligament. The posterior longitudinal ligament only affords weak reinforcement. The anterior and middle fibers are most numerous anteriorly and laterally but are deficient posteriorly where most of the fibers are attached to the cartilage plate (Fig. 1.3).

The fibers of the annulus are firmly attached to the vertebral bodies and are arranged in lamellae with the fibers of one layer running at an angle to those of the deeper layer. This anatomical arrangement permits the annulus to limit vertebral movements. This important function is reinforced by the investing vertebral ligaments. Because the nucleus pulposus is gelatinous, the load of axial compression is distributed not only in a vertical direction but radially throughout the nucleus as well. This radial distribution of the vertical load (tangential loading of the

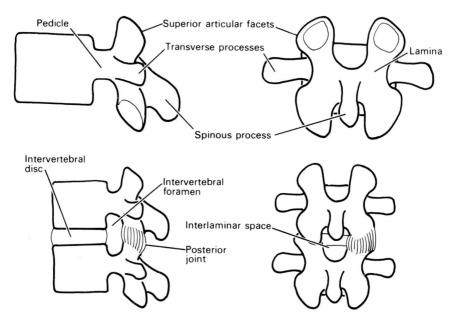

Figure 1.1.   The components of a lumbar vertebra: the body, the pedicle, the superior and inferior facets, the transverse and spinous processes, and the intervertebral foramen and its relationship to the intervertebral disc and the posterior joint.

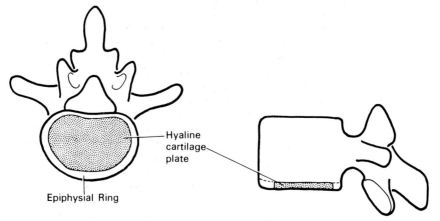

Figure 1.2.   The epiphysial ring is wider anteriorly and surrounds the hyaline cartilaginous plate.

disc) is absorbed by the fibers of the annulus (Fig. 1.4). This function of the annulus can be compared to the hoops around a barrel (Fig. 1.5).

Weight is transmitted to the nucleus through the hyaline cartilage plate. The hyaline cartilage is ideally suited to the function because it is avascular. If weight were transmitted through a vascularized structure,

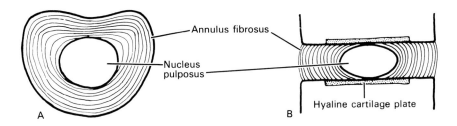

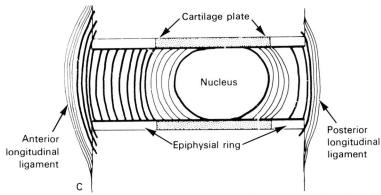

Figure 1.3. The annulus fibrosus is composed of concentric fibrous rings which surround the nucleus pulposus (*A*). The nucleus pulposus abuts against the hyaline cartilage plate (*B*). The outermost annulus fibers are most numerous anteriorly and are attached to the vertebral body immediately deep to the epiphysial ring. The epiphysial fibers run from one epiphysial ring to the other. The cartilaginous fibers run from one cartilage plate to the other cartilage plate. These comprise 90% of the annulus fibers posteriorly. The anterior fibers of the annulus are strongly reinforced by the powerful anterior longitudinal ligament, but the posterior longitudinal ligament only gives weak reinforcement to the posterior fibers of the annulus.

such as bone, the local pressure would shut off blood supply and progressive areas of bone would die. This phenomenon is seen when the cartilage plate presents congenital defects and the nucleus is in direct contact with the spongiosa of bone. The pressure occludes the blood supply, a small zone of bone dies, and the nucleus progressively intrudes into the vertebral body. This phenomenon was first described by Professor G. Schmorl and the resulting lesion bears his name, the Schmorl's node (1).

The annulus acts like a coiled spring, pulling the vertebral bodies together against the elastic resistance of the nucleus pulposus with the result that when a spine is sectioned sagittally the unopposed pull of the annulus makes the nucleus bulge. This has been referred to as "turgor" of the nucleus but, in actual fact, it is manifestation of a spring-like action, the compressing action, of the annulus fibrosus. This makes for a very good coupling unit, provided that all of the structures remain intact.

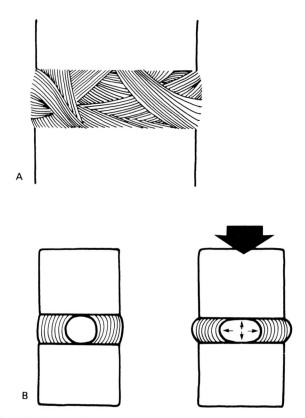

Figure 1.4. *A*, the annulus is a laminated structure with the fibrous lamellae running obliquely. This disposition of the fibers permits resistance of torsional strains. *B*, the nucleus pulposus is constrained by the fibers of the annulus. When a vertical load is applied to the vertebral column, the force is dissipated radially by the gelatinous nucleus pulposus. Distortion and disruption of the nucleus pulposus are resisted by the annulus.

The nucleus pulposus acts like a ball bearing and, in flexion and extension, the vertebral bodies roll over this incompressible gel while the posterior joints guide and steady the movements (Fig. 1.6).

The intervertebral discs have a blood supply up to the age of 8 (2), but thereafter they are dependent for their nutrition on diffusion of tissue fluids. This fluid transfer is bidirectional from vertebral body to disc and from disc to vertebral body. The ability to transfer fluid from the discs to the adjacent vertebral bodies minimizes the rise in intradiscal pressure on sudden compression loading. This fluid transfer acts like a safety valve and protects the disc. Clinical experience supported by experimental observations has shown that the fibers of the annulus are not usually ruptured by direct compression loading (3) (Fig. 1.7). Sudden severe

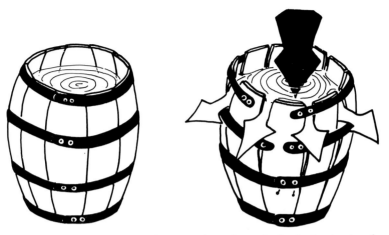

Figure 1.5. Hoop stress. This diagram shows how the load of water in a barrel is resisted by the hoops around the barrel. When too great a load is applied, the hoops will break. The annulus functions in a manner similar to the hoops around a water barrel.

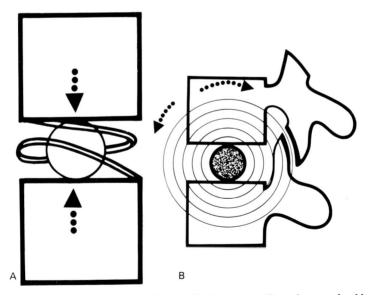

Figure 1.6. *A*, the annulus acts like a coiled spring, pulling the vertebral bodies together against the elastic resistance of the nucleus pulposus. *B*, the nucleus pulposus acts as a ball bearing with the vertebral bodies rolling over this incompressible gel in flexion and extension while the posterior joints guide and steady the movement.

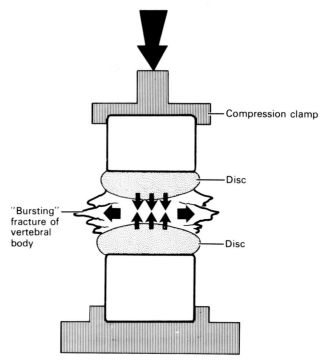

Figure 1.7. Diagram to show the experimental testing of vertical loading of the spine. When a very high compressive force is applied, the discs will remain intact but the vertebral body shatters.

loading of the spine, however, may produce a rise of fluid pressure within the vertebral body great enough to produce a "bursting" fracture.

Although this has been a very cursory review of the structure and function of the intervertebral disc, it can be seen that the components of a disc act as an integrated whole subserving many functions in addition to being a roller bearing between adjacent vertebral bodies.

The zygapophysial joints are arthrodial joints permitting simple gliding movements. Although the lax capsule of the zygapophysial joints is reinforced to some extent by the ligamentum flavum anteriorly and the supraspinous ligament posteriorly (Fig. 1.8), the major structures restraining movement in these joints are the outermost fibers of the annulus. When these fibers exhibit degenerative changes, excessive joint play is permitted. This is the reason why degenerative changes within the discs render the related posterior joints vulnerable to strain.

One of the important anatomical features of the lumbar spine is the relationship the neural elements bear to the bony skeleton and the intervertebral discs. The spinal cord ends at L1. From this point all of the lumbar, sacral, and coccygeal nerve roots run as distinct entities

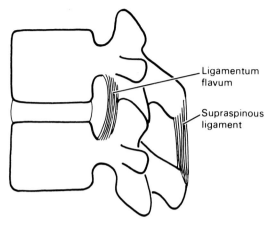

Ligamentum flavum

Supraspinous ligament

Figure 1.8. The supraspinous ligament and the ligamentum flavum must be regarded as reinforcing or accessory ligaments for the posterior zygapophysial joints.

ensheathed within the dural sac and exit through the lumbar, sacral, and coccygeal intervertebral foramina.

The clinical significance of this anatomical feature is that a tumor can involve any one of the lumbar or sacral nerves at any level in the lumbar spine canal. A tumor may selectively involve the first sacral root at the level of L3 and thereby give rise to considerable confusion in diagnosis.

The nerve roots as they leave the cauda equina course downward and outward crossing an intervertebral disc, passing anterior to the superior articular facet, and then hugging the medial aspect of the pedicle before emerging through the intervertebral foramen. At its point of emergence from the foramen, the nerve root is once again in intimate contact with the lateral posterior aspect of an intervertebral disc. The nerve root, therefore, is vulnerable to compression by pathological changes occurring at several points during its course down the spinal canal (Fig. 1.9).

In this regard variations in the configuration of the spinal canal are of special anatomical interest. The configuration of the normal spinal canal allows ample space for the contained neural elements. However, an anterior convexity of the laminae decreases the size of the spinal canal and a massive development of coronally disposed articular facets decreases the size of the "tunnel" through which the roots must pass to enter the intervertebral foramina (Fig. 1.10). In the presence of such anatomical variants, pathological changes in the discs or zygapophysial joints of relatively minor degree may produce root compromise of clinical significance.

Although the lumbar spine is a beautifully constructed multisegmental column, it must be remembered that the necessity for mobility renders it vulnerable to strain. Lucas (4) showed that the lumbar spine of a

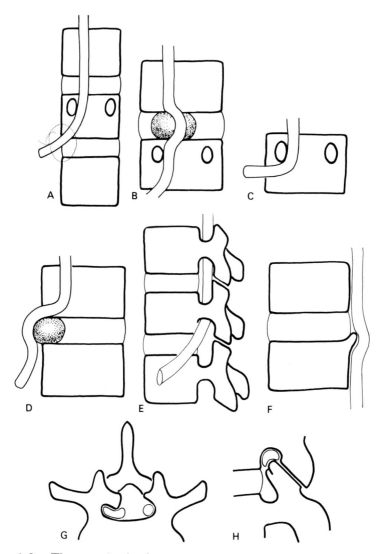

Figure 1.9. The emerging lumbar nerve roots cross over an intervertebral disc and then sweep around the pedicle before emerging through the intervertebral foramen at which point they are in contact with the lateral aspect of the disc below (*A*). It can be seen, therefore, that the nerve root can be compressed by a protrusion of the disc that it passes over (*B*); by kinking around the pedicle (*C*); and after it has emerged through the foramen by lateral protrusion of an intervertebral disc (*D*). In the lateral view it can be seen that the nerve root as it courses down to emerge through the foramen has to pass underneath the superior articular facet and across the dorsal aspect of the vertebral bodies before it emerges through the foramen (*E*). The nerve root, therefore, may be compressed by an osteophyte derived from the posterior aspect of a vertebral body (*F*), it may be compressed as it runs through the subarticular gutter (*G*), and finally it may be compressed in the foramen by the tip of a subluxated superior articular facet (*H*).

8

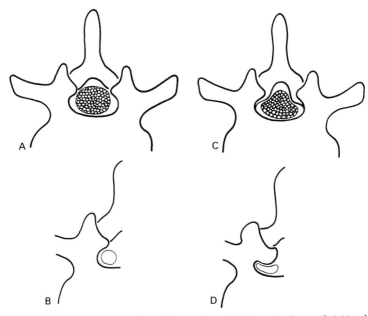

Figure 1.10. In the normal configuration of the spinal canal (*A*), there is plenty of room for the cauda equina and the emerging nerve roots to course through the subarticular gutter (*B*) without constraint. In spinal stenosis, the spinal canal assumes a trefoil shape (*C*) and this anatomical variation not only constricts the cauda equina but also narrows the tunnel through which the nerve roots must pass to enter the intervertebral foramina. When this anatomical variant is associated with hypertrophy of the posterior facets, the emerging nerve roots may be compressed as they pass along the subarticular gutter (*D*).

cadaver, dissected free from all muscular attachments, would buckle when placed under a load as small as 5 pounds. Nachemson and his co-workers (5) estimated that when an object was held 14 inches away from the spine, the load on the lumbosacral disc was 15 times the weight lifted. Lifting up a 100-pound weight at arms' length theoretically places a 1500-pound load on the lumbosacral disc.

This load must, of course, be dissipated: otherwise the fifth lumbar vertebra would crush. This load is dissipated through the paraspinal muscles and, most importantly of all, by the abdominal cavity which acts as a hydraulic chamber absorbing and diminishing the load applied.

These observations on the loading of the spine are mentioned solely to emphasize the vulnerability of the spine to the mechanical stresses placed on it by the activities of daily living, particularly in people with poor muscle tone.

Although the sacroiliac joint was regarded for many years as a common source of low back pain, its bony configuration, its limited range of movement, and its powerful ligamentous supports all serve to prevent this articulation from being vulnerable to minor injuries (Fig. 1.11).

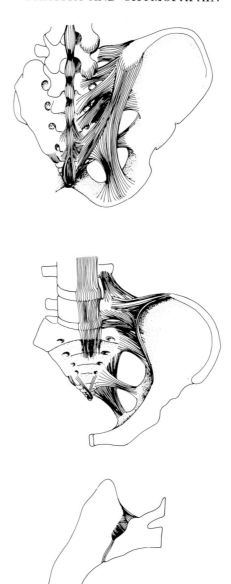

Figure 1.11. The sacroiliac joints are reinforced by very powerful ligaments both anteriorly and posteriorly in addition to the posterior interosseus ligaments. With this strong ligamentous support, the joint is indeed extremely stable, readily able to withstand the physical trauma associated with the activities of every day living.

Indeed, it is only when the ligamentous supports of the sacroiliac joint have been relaxed in the latter stages of pregnancy that injurious movements can occur without extreme violence.

This concludes our Brownian movement assault on basic anatomy principles. Most of you know this and we apologize for the insult. Further anatomical-clinical considerations are covered in Chapter 10, Technique of Chemonucleolysis.

References

1. Schmorl G, Junghanus H: *The Human Spine in Health and Disease* (Besemann EF, translator). New York, Grune & Stratton, 1971.
2. Coventry MB, Ghormley RK, Kernohan JW: The intervertebral disc: Its microscopic anatomy and pathology. *J Bone Joint Surg* 27:105, 1945.
3. Farfan HFA: A reorientation in the surgical approach to a degenerative lumbar intervertebral joint disease. *Orthop Clin North Am* 8:9, 1977.
4. Lucas DB: Mechanics of the spine. *Bull Hosp Joint Dis* 31:115, 1970.
5. Nachemson A: The load of lumbar discs in different positions of the body. *Clin Orthop* 45:107, 1966.

Epidemiological Aspects of a Herniated Nucleus Pulposus

Low back pain is a high profile symptom in industrialized societies. A study in England (1) revealed that 2% of the population annually sought medical care for back pain. Other studies (2) have shown that approximately 60% of men aged 25 to 69 have had back pain at one time or another. Under age 45, back pain is the most common cause of activity limitations (3), while over age 45 it ranks third to heart disease and arthritis. Overall, back pain is second only to the common cold as a cause of lost time from work. It is estimated that 4 hours per person per year are lost from work because of back pain (4).

One must recognize that a herniated nucleus pulposus is not the most common cause of low back pain. On the other hand, the diagnosis of a herniated nucleus pulposus is a common reason for invasive surgical considerations. A United States National Health Survey found that 1% of persons per year of age 17 to 64 had symptoms suggestive of a herniated nucleus pulposus (5) and approximately 150,000 United States patients per year undergo a simple lumbar discectomy (6).

FACTORS AFFECTING INCIDENCE OF NUCLEUS PULPOSUS HERNATION

Age

A herniated nucleus pulposus is more likely to occur between the ages of 30 to 40 years when the disc is in the process of decreasing its water content. Below the age of 30, the resilience of the disc protects it from herniation; above the age of 40, a disc has developed some degree of inherent stability through fibrous changes that occur with loss of turgor (7). Everyone has seen exceptions to this age range with younger patients and older patients presenting with the classic picture of a herniated nucleus pulposus.

Sex

Most epidemiological studies reveal a higher rate of disc prolapse in men ranging from slightly higher than 1:1 to 2:1. A multiparous woman has an increased chance of developing a nuclear prolapse.

Occupation

It would appear that those who lift, carry, pull, or push in the line of duty are *not* subject to a higher incidence of disc prolapse. People who sit more than 50% of the time have a higher incidence of nuclear prolapse. Driving a truck appears to increase the incidence of disc prolapse fourfold (8).

12

Injury

Within the Workmen's Compensation Board group of patients, 70% will report an occupational incident such as lifting as the cause of low back pain and sciatica. Outside of Compensation Board patients, half as many report an injury as the initiating event in their symptom complex.

The absence of injury as the cause of back pain and sciatica is easily explained by the natural phenomenon of aging (*cf.* Chapter 3) and the repeated torsional strains that befall the disc in upright *Homo sapiens* (*cf.* Chapter 4).

Patients who lift heavy loads and do so repeatedly do not have an increased incidence of herniated nucleus pulposus (9). This fact raises serious doubts about the cost effectiveness of numerous posters, seminars, etc., emphasizing the right and the wrong way to lift.

Habits

Height and weight appear to have little effect on the incidence of herniated nucleus pulposus (7). It is a long-standing tradition in office practice to encourage overweight patients with back disorders to lose weight, yet there is no consistent scientific study to show that this sacrifice makes any difference.

We live in a physically more active society, with encouragement from many directions to seek improved health through exercise. While this applies to such things as cardiovascular and mental well-being, there is no evidence that increased physical activity will protect one from a disc prolapse.

While good habits seem to carry little reward relative to disc prolapse, the habit of smoking and its associated respiratory tract irritation increase the chance of falling prey to back pain and sciatica due to a disc herniation (8).

Emotional State

While much is said and written about low back pain and stress, there is no body of scientific study that suggests those with emotional illness have an increased incidence of low back pain and sciatica. It is more likely that the two conditions can coexist independently for a short time, but eventually (and sometimes immediately) emotional lability will increase the degree of disability, sometimes beyond the bounds of reason.

References

1. Dillane JB, Fry J, Katon G: Acute back syndrome—A study from general practice. *Br Med J* 2:82, 1966.
2. Hult L: Cervical, dorsal, and lumbar spinal syndromes. *Acta Orthop Scand* Suppl. 17, 1954.
3. National Center for Health Statistics: *Limitation of Activity Due to Chronic Conditions, United States 1969 and 1970.* Series 10, Number 80, 1973.
4. Rowe ML: Low back pain in industry. A position paper. *J Occup Med* 11:161, 1969.

5. National Center for Health Statistics: *Prevalence of Chronic Skin and Musculo-Skeletal Conditions, United States, 1969.* Series 10, Number 92, 1974.
6. Commission on Professional Hospital Activity of Ann Arbor, Michigan: *Hospital Records Study.* Ambler, PA, IMS America Ltd., 1978.
7. Kelsey JL, White AA: Epidemiology and impact of low-back pain. *Spine* 5:133, 1980.
8. Frymoyer J, Pope MH, Costanza MC, *et al*: Epidemiologic studies of low back pain. *Spine* 5:419, 1980.
9. Kelsey JL: An epidemiological study of the relationship between occupations and acute herniated lumbar intervertebral discs. *Int J Epidemiol* 4:197, 1975.

CHAPTER 3

Biological Basis of a Herniated Nucleus Pulposus

The basic element of a living organism is the cell (protoplasm) made up of a nucleus and cytoplasm. The cell can nourish itself, grow, respond to stimuli, and reproduce. Cells group together, surround themselves with various types and amounts of fiber support, and embed themselves in amorphous background material (extracellular substance, ground substance, or matrix) to form tissues.

The basic medium in which the protoplasmic constituents of tissues are dispersed is water. Both inside and outside the cell, the water combines with soluble organic molecules and salts to form a colloid mass. This viscid mass varies its fluid consistency by varying the type and amount of cells, fiber, and ground substance.

The four basic macromolecules that allow for this variation are: nucleic acid, proteins, complex carbohydrates, and lipids.

Of the four basic adult tissues (epithelium, contractile, neural, and connective), the intervertebral disc is classified as a dense fibrocartilaginous connective tissue. To grasp its response to the injection of a proteolytic enzyme such as chymopapain, it is essential to understand the biochemistry of the protein and carbohydrate macromolecules and their various combinations.

Proteins are the building blocks of cells and tissues. The basic unit of protein is amino acid, of which approximately 20 varieties exist in living systems. Through various sequences and numbers, these amino acids join, through peptide bonds, to form a particular protein.

Proteins can be classified according to the shape they take or the company they keep. The molecule of protein may be a single or multiple peptide chain (such as insulin) or, through additional bonding, the chains can coil on themselves to produce the helical arrangement of collagen. Unaccompanied proteins (such as albumin and globulin) are known as simple proteins and yield only amino acids on hydrolysis. The proteins we are interested in are conjugated with polymers of sugars known as mucopolysaccharides or glycosaminoglycans. The complex protein-polysaccharide molecule thus formed constitutes 50% of dry weight of nucleus polposus and is called a proteoglycan.

STRUCTURE OF LUMBAR INTERVERTEBRAL DISC

Three distinct tissues constitute the intervertebral disc—nucleus pulposus, annulus fibrosis, and two hyaline cartilage end plates. The disc has evolved to allow for movement between vertebral bodies and to absorb forces transferred through the axial skeleton.

The annulus is made up predominantly of coarse collagen fibers in sheets or lamellae of parallel fibers that interconnect adjacent vertebral

15

bodies and end plates. The lamellae are concentrically arranged around a central nucleus with fibers in each lamellae lying in a different direction to its adjacent lamellae (1) to form a lattice like a Japanese finger trap (*cf.* Chapter 1, Figs. 1.3 and 1.4). The lamellae slip over each other during movement and stress through a viscoelastic slippage inherent in the biochemical makeup of the annular fissures.

A transitional zone of fiber and ground substance exists between the annulus and nucleus which blends with the gelatinous central core of nucleus pulposus (made up of loosely distributed collagen and abundant ground substance).

The cells of the annulus and nucleus are variously classified as chondrocytes or fibrocytes and are derived from mesenchymal stem cells. Although embryonic notocord cells are present in the nucleus, it is felt they are not the source of all the cells in the nucleus.

The extracellular substance or matrix of the disc is a combination of collagen, proteoglycans, and H_2O. The outer annulus is the most collagenous and the inner nucleus the least collagenous. The fibrous network of collagen is responsible for the strength of the disc. Normal adults appear to have a lower content of collagen in the posterolateral part of the annulus fibrosus, the usual site for disc herniations. The proteoglycan gradient is reversed from nucleus to annulus with only 50% of the nucleus, by dry weight content, being collagen.

The collagen of the disc is divided into type I and type II according to molecular composition (2). Type II collagen is more prevalent in bone, tendon, and skin. Both types are present in the disc with type I concentration higher in the periphery of the annulus and type II becoming more prevalent as you move towards the transitional zone. Overall, type II makes up 60% of the disc substance.

Proteoglycans constitute 10% of the dry weight of the outer annulus and 50% of dry weight of the nucleus pulposus. After H_2O and collagen, they are the third most abundant component of the normal intervertebral disc. Their major function is to keep the fibrous framework or the cartilage pressurized with retained water, such that the disc is able to resist and distribute compressive forces. Their biochemistry is a protein core with polysaccharide side chains (glycosaminoglycans). The major glycosaminoglycans of annulus fibrosus and nucleus pulposus are chondroitin sulfate and keratin sulfate. Through their sulfated structure, the proteoglycans have a negative charge.

A fourth constituent (macromolecule) of the disc is glycoprotein (or mucoprotein). This noncollagenous protein is bound to fibrils and probably plays a role in regulating fiber thickness, quality, and strength of interaction with proteoglycans and H_2O content of ground substance.

NUTRITION, METABOLISM, AND AGING

There are no blood vessels present in the adult disc. Thus, nutritional supply for the disc must come through the ligaments that sheath the periphery of the disc and the vascular beds that lie in the subchondral area of the vertebral body adjacent to the porous cartilaginous end plate of disc. Nachemson and co-workers (3) feel that physiochemical differences determine that uncharged molecules like glucose and oxygen enter the disc mainly via the end plates. Charged molecules like sulfate ions, important for glucosaminoglycan production, enter mainly via the annulus fibrosus. With aging, there is a decrease in the rate of nutrient diffusion to the nucleus pulposus and annulus. This interferes with synthesis of collagen and proteoglycans resulting in a "drying out" of the disc (loss of H_2O content).

At this stage there is a relative increase in collagen and a disappearance of ground substance in the nucleus. The change in collagen volume is accompanied with broader fiber bundles.

Because nutritional requirements are not met, the nucleus solidifies and its efficiency in distributing stresses from vertical and torsional loads declines. With this, the physical appearance of cracks and crevices occurs and the process of disc degeneration is on its way.

References

1. Eyre DR: *Biochemistry of the Intervertebral Disc*, International Review of Connective Tissue Research, Vol. 8. New York, Academic Press, 1979.
2. Naylor A, Happey F, Turner RL, *et al*: Enzymatic and immunologic activity in the intervertebral disc. *Orthop Clin North Am* 6:51, 1975.
3. Nachemson A, Lewin T, Maroudas A, *et al*: In vitro diffusion of dye through the end plates and the annulus fibrosus of human lumbar intervertebral discs. *Acta Orthop Scand* 41:589, 1970.

CHAPTER 4

Biomechanical Concepts in Herniated Nucleus Pulposus

Nutritional changes in proteins and the resulting alteration in the histochemical makeup of a disc cannot explain, by themselves, how nuclear material herniates through a rent in the annulus. Further explanation for nuclear protrusions comes through an understanding of the movement forces applied to a normal and abnormal (degenerated) spinal motion segment.

Movement forces applied to the axial skeleton are absorbed and dissipated through the special hydrostatic nature of the disc. The fluid nature of the nuclear gel allows for absorption of forces and the intimate contact between nucleus and annulus allows for dissipation of these loads into the elastic coil structure of the annulus. Further support for this force transmission is found in the various ligaments and muscles attached to processes, body, and posterior arch of the vertebral segment.

Abnormal nuclear movement or disc failure can occur in one of three ways.

a. Nuclear material may herniate through the end plate (a Schmorl's node).

b. Nuclear-annular integrity can be altered from within resulting in a progressive disruption of annular integrity from within, towards the outer boundary of the annulus.

c. Annular integrity can be altered from without, when forces applied to the motion segment exceed the normal resistance of the annulus, cleaving the outer fibers. With further injury, this rent extends inward to eventually communicate with the nucleus and create a path for nuclear migration.

There are numerous forces that can be applied, alone or in combination, to a spinal segment. Complex mathematical equations (1) are used to describe the resulting distortion of the disc architecture. For the purpose of this monograph a simple concept of only three forces, acting singly, will be considered.

COMPRESSION

Discs can be subjected to very high compressive loads. These forces increase the pressure within the nucleus (2) and result in a minor loss (5%) of nuclear water with a decrease in volume of the nucleus. Further absorption of the force occurs through bulging of the annulus. In normal discs this increased annular fiber tension results in increased angulation in the collagen lamellar pattern. With increasing compression in a normal disc, the nuclear pressure and annular tension changes will sustain until the end plate fails (1500 to 2000 pounds)—the so-called "end plate

18

fracture." As mentioned, this herniation of nuclear material through the end plate and the subsequent healing of bone has a characteristic appearance on x-ray of a Schmorl's node.

With alteration of the nucleus-annulus junction through aging, repeated compressive loads may initiate annular fissures from within the disc. Eventually nuclear material may protrude part way through the annulus, but still be enclosed by the annulus. This nuclear material creates a localized bulge in the annulus, which in turn may compromise an adjacent nerve root (Fig. 4.1). On discography this disc will be contained (Fig. 4.2) (*cf.* Chapter 10).

TORSION

Experimental evidence would suggest that torsion, along with bending, is the most damaging force applied to a disc (3). The application of torsion (twisting or rotating on the long axis) produces tensile and shear stresses in the annulus. These forces are greatest on the outermost fibers

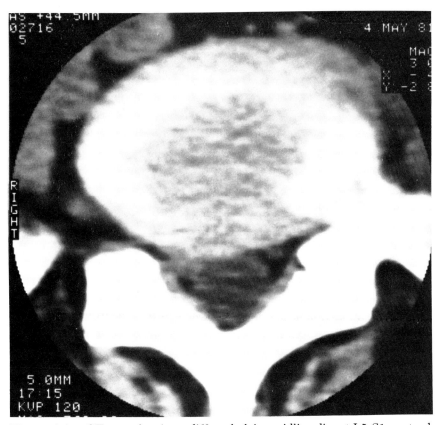

Figure 4.1. CT scan showing a diffuse, bulging midline disc at L5-S1, protruding more to the right.

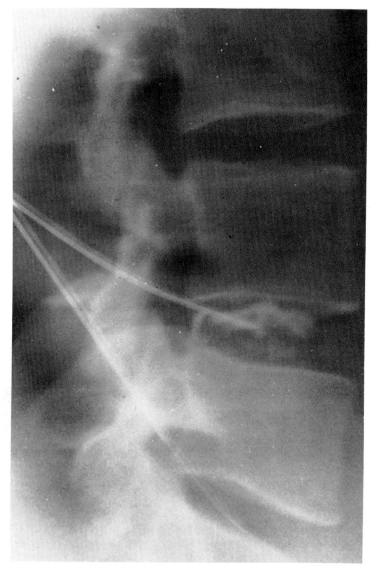

Figure 4.2.   Discogram (L4-5) showing contrast material extending to posterior annular region but still "contained" within the annulus.

of the annulus and decrease as one moves towards the center of the disc where very little force is applied to the nucleus. In addition, the facet joints may be damaged by absorbing some of these torsional strains. At times the facet joints are damaged by torsion to the point where the vertebral segment is permanently rotated. Farfan believes this rotation can compress the root because the medial migration of the pedicle may kink the existing nerve root and, in such instances, the resulting myelographic defect may mimic a disc herniation.

A forced rotational injury will damage the annulus but not the end plates. This is because the force is greatest on the outer annular fibers and it is here that the first radial fissures start. With repeated torsional strains, the radial fissure will work its way inward, ultimately connecting with the nuclear cavity forming a pathway through which nuclear material can extrude.

The posterolateral portions of the annulus are thinner and weaker than the rest of the annulus, and it is here that a torsion stress has its maximal effect. Further alteration in the localization of these stress risers comes through the shape of the posterior vertebral border to which the annulus is attached. The "rounder" the shape (L5-S1), the closer the stress riser is to the midline. The "flatter" the shape (L4-5), the more lateral will be the stress riser and resulting annular damage.

About 95% of nuclear protrusions will occur at L4-5 and L5-S1. Younger patients tend to have an increased incidence of disc herniation at the L5-S1 level because stress increases at the junction of mobility (L5) and fixation (S1 and pelvis). With slow aging and degeneration, an inherent stability will develop in the L5-S1 disc through loss of turgor and elasticity, with subsequent fibrosis of the disc. This transfers more stress to the level above, explaining the higher incidence of nuclear protrusion at the L4-5 level that occurs with increasing age.

Further protection of the L5-S1 disc segment from torsion stress occurs when L5 is set low in the pelvis on S1 or when L5 has a long transverse process (and thus a short iliolumbar ligament). This built-in stability of L5 on S1 offers protection from rotational forces and transfers the stress riser to the L4-5 disc. (Fig. 4.3).

BENDING

Bending has occurred when the upper surface of a disc tilts in respect to its lower surface. As with torsion stresses, there is very little increase in nuclear pressure and thus no end plate failure occurs. However, forward bending will cause increased tension (stretch) on posterior annular fibers and may cause failure of the annulus in this area. Compression and torsion distribute forces evenly around the cross-section of a disc while forward bending localizes forces to the posterior collagenous fibers. This bending can have a very disruptive effect on the posterior annulus, cleaving the annulus or separating the annular fibers from the vertebral body or end plate. As with torsion injury, these annular disruptions can extend to nuclear territory and create a pathway for nuclear herniation.

SUMMARY

It is obvious that nuclear migration through the annulus represents a combined effect of aging, with molecular alteration of the nucleus pulposus and annulus fibrosus, and repeated mechanical stresses to the

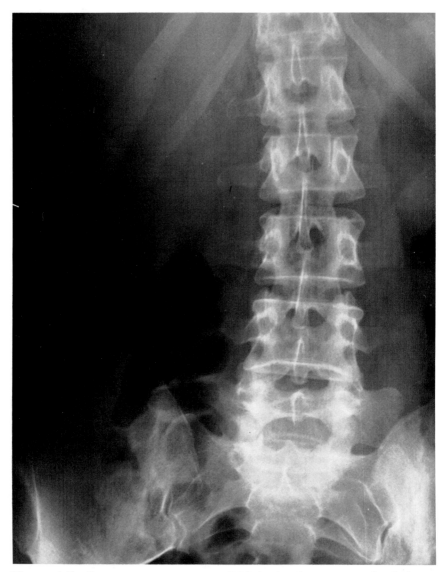

Figure 4.3.   Large transverse process, L5 left, that increases mechanical stability at L5-S1, and transfers stress riser to L4-5.

motion segment. No one cause of disc herniation can be pinpointed. This explains, to some extent, the many different clinical combinations of symptoms, signs, and investigative findings confronting the clinician when making the diagnosis of a herniated nucleus pulposus.

References

1. Hickey DS, Hakins DWL: Relation between the structure of the annulus fibrosus and the function and failure of the intervertebral disc. *Spine* 5:106, 1980.
2. Nachemson A: The lumbar spine. An orthopedic challenge. *Spine* 1:59, 1976.
3. Farfan HFA: A reorientation in the surgical approach to degenerative lumbar intervertebral joint disease. *Orthop Clin North Am* 8:9, 1977.

CHAPTER 5

The Pathogenesis of Sciatica

Sciatica is pain radiating down the posterior aspect of the leg in the distribution of the sciatic nerve. Associated may be symptoms of paresthesia (numbness, tingling, pins, and needles) or weakness. Anterior thigh pain is called "anterior crural" pain and is derived from femoral nerve lesions.

Sciatic pain, or leg pain mimicking sciatica, may arise from several sources. The most common is radicular pain from nerve root tension, irritation, and/or compression from disc material, or osseous encroachment on the canal or lateral recess. Root compression or irritation may also be derived from benign or malignant extradural or intrathecal tumors. The intermittent claudication of peripheral vascular disease may mimic radicular pain in a sciatic distribution (Table 5.1).

REFERRED PAIN

The major factor that has clouded and confused the diagnosis of the sources of sciatica is the phenomenon of referred pain. When a deep structure is irritated either by trauma or disease, the pain resulting may be experienced locally, referred distally or proximally, or experienced both locally and radiating to a distance. For example, pain asociated with a cyst of the lateral meniscus may radiate proximally and distally in a sciatic distribution. The presence and distribution of referred pain can be demonstrated by the experimental injection of the supraspinous ligament between L5 and S1 (1) (Fig. 5.1).

The mechanism of referred pain is beyond the scope of this monograph. Suffice it to say that segmental instability secondary to disc degeneration alone at L4-5 and L5-S1 may, on occasion, give rise to acute or chronic low back pain associated with pain radiating down the leg in a sciatic distribution. Referred pain due to L4-5 segmental instability is frequently referred to the anterosuperior iliac spine region or groin and from L5-S1 to the anterior thigh region.

REMEMBER—Referred pain 1) rarely radiates below the knee, 2) is often bilateral, 3) is more vague than radicular pain due to sciatic nerve root involvement, and 4) is not associated with paresthesia.

On examination, patients with segmental instability may, during an acute episode, have a "locked back" with marked limitation of both flexion and extension of the spine. With the patient lying supine on the examination table, passive straight leg raising is usually permitted to 60° or above and the pain is not aggravated by popliteal pressure or forced dorsiflexion of the ankle. When bilateral active straight leg raising is performed, the weight of the legs tend to rotate the pelvis, thereby hyperextending the lumbosacral junction. If a patient is suffering from degenerative disc change, bilateral active straight leg raising will invoke a painful response in the back.

Table 5.1.
Differential Diagnosis of Sciatica

A. INTRASPINAL CAUSES
    1. Proximal to disc—conus and cauda equina lesions (*e.g.*, neurofibroma, ependymoma)
    2. Disc level—herniated nucleus pulposus
                —stenosis (canal or recess)
                —infection (osteomyelitis, discitis)
                —inflammation (arachnoiditis)
                —neoplasm (benign, malignant)
                    (bone, nonbone)
B. EXTRASPINAL CAUSES
    1. Pelvis—cardiovascular conditions (*e.g.*, aorto-iliac disease, thrombophlebitis)
                —gynecological conditions (*e.g.*, endometriosis)
                —orthopaedic conditions (*e.g.*, osteoarthritis hip, torn lateral meniscus)
                —SI joint disease
                —metastases to bone
    2. Peripheral nerve lesions—neuropathy (diabetic, alcoholic, tumor)
                          —conditions local to sciatic nerve (trauma, tumors)
C. MISCELLANEOUS—Nonorganic

Neurological examination of the lower extremities does not reveal any evidence of root irritation, root tension, or impairment of root conduction. In the absence of any evidence of any form of compromise of the cauda equina or lumbar nerve roots, there is very little justification, if any, for performing a myelogram. Occasionally, a "desperation" diagnostic myelogram is performed. Unfortunately, this may show a "defect" in the radiopaque column. The small myelographic defect is usually at the level of L4-5 (Fig. 5.2). On the anteroposterior view, the defect is bilateral and gives rise to the picture of a narrowing or wasting of the "oil column." On the lateral view, there may be an anterior indentation of the contrast material. It is to be noted that these "deceptive defects" are more likely to be seen with oil-soluble myelography than with metrizamide.

This type of radiographic defect is due to a diffuse annular bulge of the disc. If an "exploratory" laminotomy is performed, it can be seen that the root is *not* under tension. The nerve root can be displaced medially 1 cm and distally 0.5 cm. Obviously with this degree of mobility, the nerve root is not compromised and the disc, although demonstrating a diffuse annular bulge, would not be productive of root compression. The leg pain in these patients is *referred* pain due to segmental instability. Discectomy may increase the instability and could aggravate the symptoms. Chemonucleolysis decompression will also fail to relieve symptoms.

In this group of patients, if despite adequate conservative treatment the patient's pain is of sufficient severity to prevent the patient from continuing his work and prevent him from enjoying his leisure hours, then surgery may be considered. Surgical intervention, however, must be designed to overcome segmental instability and the patient will require

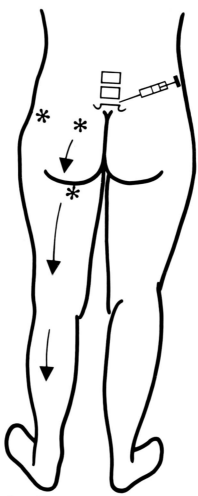

Figure 5.1. The injection of hypertonic saline into the supraspinous ligament between L5 and S1 will give rise to local pain and pain referred down the back of the leg in sciatic distribution. In addition to this, there will be areas of tenderness produced in the lower limb most commonly at the sites noted by the *asterisks.*

a spinal fusion—not a discectomy. *Neither chemonucleolysis nor discectomy has any place in the treatment of patients with discogenic segmental instability associated with referred pain in a sciatic distribution.*

In 1934, Mixter and Barr (2) suggested that sciatic pain could result from irritation of the lumbar nerve root by a prolapsed intervertebral disc.

Although skeptically received at first, this concept soon became universally accepted and founded the *"dynasty of the disc"*—during which time the complaint of sciatic pain tended to become uncritically equated

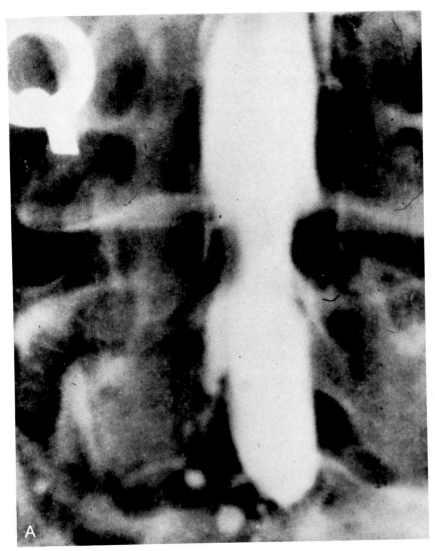

Figure 5.2. *A*, the typical waisting or hourglass constriction of the oil column associated with a diffuse annular bulge, commonly seen with degenerative segmental stenosis. *B*, myelogram showing shallow L4-5 defect. The discogram at this level was normal.

with a diagnosis of a disc rupture. The term "ruptured disc" was soon used so loosely that it lost much of its clinical significance and indeed there has been a profusion and confusion of terminology. Sometimes the operative note would state with disarming simplicity: "a disc was found." The height of absurdity was the introduction of the term, "concealed disc" (3), to describe a ruptured disc which would not be demonstrated at operation. Surgeons forgot that a ruptured disc gave rise to symptoms

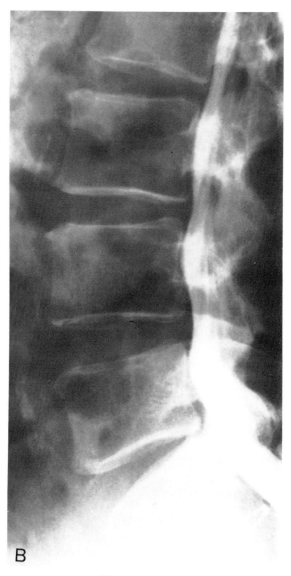

Figure 5.2B.

solely by producing nerve root pressure. They forgot that all the surgeon can state, on clinical examination, is that the patient is suffering from root compromise. This is an important basic concept: the surgeon can only diagnose root compromise. There is no specific clinical sign that irrefutably indicates that the root pressure from which the patient is suffering is due to a prolapsed disc.

In an attempt to avoid the confusion of terminology, it is suggested that the following classification be considered (4). Disc ruptures can be defined as a distortion of the normal anatomical configuration of the annulus. Two major anatomical lesions can be distinguished: disc protrusions and disc herniations:

a. Disc protrusion
b. Disc extrusion   ⎫
c. Disc sequestration   ⎬   Disc herniations or disc ruptures
                        ⎭

DISC PROTRUSIONS

Normally the annulus fibrosus forms a smooth continuous ring confining the nucleus pulposus. On occasion, following degenerative changes, a portion of the annulus fibrosus may give way and a localized bulge occurs even though the annulus fibers are still intact (*cf.* Chapter 4).

With disc collapse, the annulus circumferentially protrudes beyond the peripheral rim of the vertebral bodies. The appearance is as though the disc has been made of putty and the vertebral bodies have been compressed together, "the middle age spread of a middle-aged disc." In disc protrusions, the distortion of the annulus may be a localized annular bulge or a diffuse annular bulge. In both instances, *the annular fibers remain intact* and at operation, when a square window is cut in the annulus, the nucleus may or may not spontaneously extrude.

DISC HERNIATIONS

Disruptions of the annular fibers permit extrusion or sequestration of the nucleus. Following detachment of a segment of the cartilage plate and/or disruption of the posterior annular fibers, a portion of the annulus may be displaced posteriorly. Beneath this the nucleus follows the displaced segment, and some nuclear material may be forced through the break in the annular fibers. Two types can be recognized, depending on the extent of displacement of nuclear material (Fig. 5.3).

To summarize:
a. *Protruded Intervertebral Disc*
   The displaced nuclear material is confined solely by a few of the outermost fibers of the annulus. At operation a discreet prominence of the annulus can be demonstrated, and when this is incised and nuclear material sometimes spontaneously extrudes through the incision.
b. *Extruded Intervertebral Disc*
   In this lesion, the displaced nuclear material has burst through the posterior fibers of the annulus and lies under the posterior investing ligament. On incising this thin ligament, the extruded fragment can be recognized and picked up with forceps. As it is withdrawn from the wound, it can be seen that the tail of the fragment was lying in a defect of the annulus.
c. *Sequestered Intervertebral Disc*
   Nuclear material may be extruded through the posterior fibers of the annulus and through the posterior longitudinal ligament. *The fragment lies free in the spinal canal.* An extruded disc may therefore be asso-

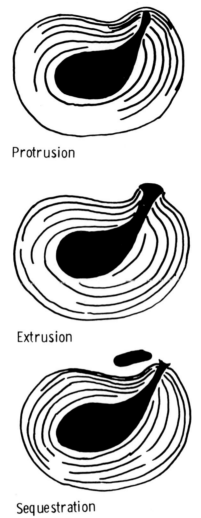

Protrusion

Extrusion

Sequestration

Figure 5.3. Stages of nuclear migration beyond the normal confines of the annulus.

ciated with a sequestrated fragment which may remain trapped between the nerve root and the annulus, while the free fragment may migrate. The sequestrated fragment may come to lie behind the vertebral body above or below the disc, in the axilla of the nerve root, in the intervertebral foramen, or in the midline anterior to the dural sac.

On occasion, the freed portion of the disc may erode or burst through the dura or even into the root sleeve.

The sequestrated portion of the disc varies in size from a small fragment attached to the apex of the extrusion, like a plume from an active volcano, to a massive segment of disc up to 20 ml in volume.

Of equal importance to the location of the disc fragment, is the nature of the fragment: a sequestered disc is often a firm mass of predominantly collagenous material (which theoretically should be unaffected by chymopapain).

d. *Intradiscal Rupture*

This is largely a theoretical concept. It is believed that on occasions the innermost fibers of the annulus will rupture, with degeneration of nuclear material producing an autoimmune reaction within the disc space. This distention within the nuclear space may produce pain.

MECHANISM OF SYMPTOM PRODUCTION DUE TO A DISC RUPTURE

There is no clear, single explanation as to why a disc rupture causes sciatica. Some disc ruptures remain asymptomatic. On routine screening of the lumbar spine when cervical myelography is performed, 5% of patients were shown to have a significant defect in the lumbar spine (5). Most myelographic defects were at L4-5 and all were asymptomatic.

In trying to understand the back and leg complaints of a patient with a herniated nucleus pulposus (HNP), a few things are clear; the patient's major complaint is pain, and physical pressure on a peripheral nerve does not produce pain, it produces paresthesia.

It is likely that no one neuromechanical theory can explain the mechanism of symptom production in an HNP. In the routine consideration of simple sciatica, seven points need to be kept in mind:

1. The description of sciatica from patient to patient is so variable that there are obviously many factors involved in the production of symptoms.
2. In the early phases of a disc herniation (a few hours to a few days), a patient may report only back pain immediately after the "snap" sensation heralding the disc rupture. During this time leg pain is absent as a symptom, root tension (straight leg raising reduction) is present as a sign, and the myelogram, if done, will be positive.
3. Some patients in the early phases of sciatica will report only paresthesia, giving rise to an irritating, diffuse, ill-localized numbness in the lower leg and foot.
4. It has been well documented (5) that patients undergoing myelography, after bed rest has successfully relieved sciatica, may still have a positive myelogram. This phenomenon has been reported up to 15 months after sciatica has disappeared.
5. In some patients undergoing successful chemonucleolysis, the CT scan defect has persisted (6) in spite of relief of symptoms and recovery from nerve root tension and compression (Fig. 5.4, *A* and *B*).
6. We have all seen the infrequent patient who notices the sudden onset of severe leg pain, quickly followed by a profound neurological lesion (*e.g.*, drop foot) followed by an equally dramatic disappearance of pain

and root tension in a few hours to a few days. Prolonged observation of these patients often reveals significant degrees of neurological recovery.

7. Pain is an unpleasant emotional state: so much depends on past experience of the patient and his emotional state and needs at the time of discomfort (*cf.* Chapter 7).

In examining this problem further, at the conclusion of a routine laminectomy for an HNP, a Fogarty catheter was placed underneath the emerging nerve root of a segment that had been decompressed and also underneath the normal nerve root at the segment above. When the patients had recovered consciousness and before they had been given any analgesics, the catheters were distended. It was found that, although distention of the catheter underneath an involved, angry red, inflamed nerve root reproduced the sciatic pain, distention of the catheter underneath the normal nerve root produced paresthesia only.

In trying to understand the mechanism of symptom production and the symptom of sciatica, we have to think of three main factors:

1. The nature of the herniated nucleus around the nerve structure.
2. Where, on the root-ganglion, the compromise is occurring.
3. Where and what is the leg symptom.

The Nature of the Herniated Nuclear Fragment

Three subfactors need to be considered: 1) mass of nuclear material, 2) distention (by proteoglycan and water) within the mass, and 3) inflammation between the mass and nerve root (Fig. 5.5).

As evidenced by the human experiment with the Fogarty catheter, the simple presence of a mass is not enough to produce sciatica. If the mass is present long enough then it will set up an inflammatory reaction which in turn produces sciatica (7).

A further consideration is the distention within the mass. If you had your choice between a cotton ball or a hard golf ball pressing on your nerve root, you would surely pick the former because of the softness and diffuseness of the pressure. However, distend the mass with proteoglycans binding the edema of inflammation and in your mind, you can just feel the pain increasing. We have had occasions to expose a large disc protrusion and noted the glistening sheen of distention present. We have then injected these discs with chymopapain, prior to annular incision, and the sheen of distention immediately disappears and the mass of disc protrusion, although still present, is obviously less distended and softer on palpation. Further, we have a number of documented cases following chemonucleolysis where symptoms and signs have been totally relieved, yet a mass still persists on CT scan (Fig. 5.4). This is no different than the persistence of a myelographic defect reported by Falconer *et al.* (5) 25 years ago and represents the "cotton ball" mass compression of a nerve root, which may be minor enough not to cause symptoms.

Thus, we may theorize that varying degrees of mass, distention, and inflammation may produce varying presentations of sciatic pain. The theoretical considerations do not stop here.

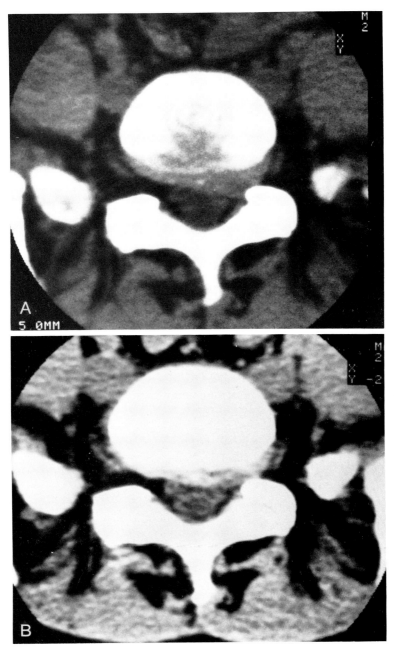

Figure 5.4. *A,* a young woman with classic sciatica, whose preinjection scan showed a large HNP at L5-S1. *B,* 3 months postinjection, the patient is pain-free and has recovered neurologically. The scan still shows a mass of HNP which is smaller.

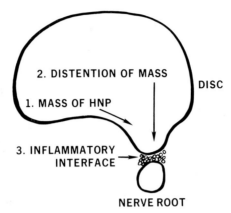

Figure 5.5. Schematic representation of the three local symptom-producing factors of an HNP.

The Location (on the Root-Ganglion) of the Lesion

The anatomical locations of pressure on an HNP are: 1) cauda equina; 2) single root, motor or sensory; 3) sympathetic fibers; and 4) dorsal root-ganglion.

The nerve tissues in the region of a disc may be compressed from the midline to the interforaminal region. Thus, roots (motor and/or sensory), ganglia, and sympathetic fibers may be the recipients of ruptured disc pressure. The pathology produced in the nervous tissue may be inflammation, edema, intraneural fibrosis, demyelination, and axonal degeneration with or without partial regeneration (5).

Where and What Is the Leg Symptom?

When considering sciatica, think of five different areas: the back, the buttock, the thigh, the calf, and the foot. There may be symptoms in all five areas or only a few of these areas.

THE BACK

Included in this area are the midline lumbosacral area, the sacroiliac joint region, the posterosuperior iliac spine, the high iliac crest area, and the low midline sacrococcygeal region. The lumbosacral region is the area where pain is often originally felt. From there, referral to the other areas may occur, the patient describing the sensation as a mechanical sharp pain that leaves the back with a fragile, unstable sensation, *i.e.*, any movement suddenly and severely increases the pain to the point where the legs may buckle or the back will "give."

THE BUTTOCK

This area should be considered the proximal extent of the leg. Pain in the middle of the buttock is to be separated from the above mentioned areas and is indicative of root interference: a) root tension, b) root irritation, and c) root compression. The pain is deep and cramp-like.

THE THIGH

Pain in this area tends to be the sharpest component of sciatica and sometimes is described as having an associated superficial "burning-sensitive" feeling. It is posterior thigh and not lateral thigh in location.

Unless the patient has a very sensitive bowstring sign, pain is usually absent from the popliteal fossa region.

THE CALF

The sensation in this area can be mixed. The prevailing discomfort is a cramp and an almost vise-like feeling in the belly of the gastrocsoleus or peroneal muscles. In addition the patient may report paresthesia in the lateral calf (fifth root) or back of the calf (first root). Most, but not all, patients with sciatica due to a herniated nucleus pulposus will have pain below the knee. The authors have seen some patients, although infrequently, with pain in the buttock and thigh only who have a proven HNP.

THE FOOT

Unlike the calf, the most common symptom in the foot is paresthesia involving the lateral border or undersurface of the foot with first sacral root involvement and the dorsum of the foot with fifth lumbar root involvement. Infrequently the patient will complain of pain in the foot, e.g., the belly of the extensor brevis muscle.

Patients with symptoms due to a HNP may have all five or some of these components of sciatica. The most common of the five areas to be free of symptoms is the back, leaving all the discomfort reported by the patient in the buttock and leg.

IT IS IMPORTANT TO EMPHASIZE HOW VARIABLE SCIATICA CAN BE AS A SYMPTOM.

Considering that a) there are motor, sensory, and sympathetic fibers, or the dorsal root ganglion, which migrated nuclear material may compress, b) the effect of an HNP on a nerve root can be compression, tension, or inflammation, separately or together, and c) with time the pathological changes in a nerve root can be inflammation, edema, intraneural fibrosis, demyelination, axonal degeneration, and regeneration, it is easy to understand that there is no one theory to explain the cause of sciatica, nor is there one classic presentation of sciatica. *Sciatica due to an HNP has many faces.*

A combination of compression, tension, and inflammation by an HNP, applied over a length of time, produces pathological changes in nerve tissue resulting in alteration in the neurophysiological functioning of the neural pathways.

These three mechanisms when applied to a sensory root will cause repetitive firing in the sensory fibers of the injured root producing the sharp pain and paresthesia of sciatica.

When applied to motor fibers, impulses to the motor segment are altered to produce a deep cramping sensation in a muscle belly.

Irritation of sympathetic fibers laterally may produce sensations of coldness in the extremity.

All of these sensations are usually aggravated by movement and relieved by rest. If there is a significant inflammatory component associated with the HNP, rest will have to be prolonged (in terms of days) before there is any relief of discomfort.

NON-NUCLEAR COMPRESSION OF NERVE ROOTS

A ruptured intervertebral disc is not the only cause of root irritation in association with disc degeneration in the lumbar spine. Others (8, 9) gradually made clinicians aware of the fact that bony overgrowth in the lumbar spinal canal or lateral recess can produce compression of the emerging nerve roots. Verbiest (8) coined the term "spinal stenosis." Soon, like the earlier dynasty of the disc, this diagnosis became indiscriminantly employed as a pathology garbage can to describe the pathogenesis of any form of leg pain not attributable to a disc rupture.

It is very important to define and discuss the bony root entrapment syndromes because these lesions are not susceptible to treatment by chemonucleolysis.

Spinal stenosis is defined as a narrowing of the spinal canal which *may* produce a bony constriction of the cauda equina and the emerging nerve roots. This bony encroachment *may* in turn produce symptoms.

The bony constraints can be considered anatomically as being either lateral giving rise to compression of the emerging nerve roots, or midline giving rise to compression of the cauda equina, or both simultaneously. These constraints may be congenital (developmental) or acquired in origin. Most cases are probably a combination of the two etiologies.

Bony compression of the emerging nerve roots arises as a result of subarticular entrapment, pedicular kinking, or foraminal impingement due to posterior joint subluxation.

Subarticular Entrapment

The nerve roots course downward and outward, passing underneath the medial border of the superior articular facets before they swing around the pedicle to emerge through the foramen. Hypertrophy of the superior articular facet may compress the nerve root between the facet and the dorsal aspect of the vertebral body (Fig. 5.6).

Pedicular Kinking

When advanced intervertebral disc degeneration is associated with marked narrowing of the disc, the vertebral bodies approach one another. As the upper vertebral body descends, its pedicle may on occasion kink the emerging nerve root to a significant degree if an asymmetrical collapse of the disc occurs (Fig. 5.7). Commonly, however, the nerve root is seen to be compressed in a gutter formed by a diffuse lateral bulge of the disc and the pedicle above (Fig. 5.8).

Foraminal Encroachment

As the root emerges through the foramen, it lies in close relation to the tip of the superior facet of the vertebra below. As the intervertebral disc narrows, the posterior joint overrides and the root may, on occasion, be compressed by the superior articular facet (Fig. 5.9).

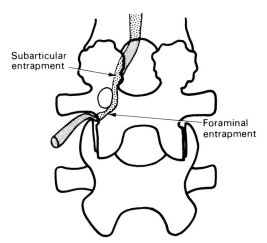

Figure 5.6.   In apophysial stenosis an emerging nerve root may be compressed at two sites. For example, as in this diagram, it may be compressed as it passes through the subarticular gutter and it may also be trapped in the foramen by the tip of the superior articular facet.

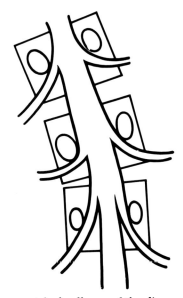

Figure 5.7.   With asymmetrical collapse of the disc and tilting of the vertebral body, the nerve root may be kinked by the pedicle giving rise to severe compression.

Midline Compression

Midline compression may be a sequel of disc degeneration when, following narrowing of the intervertebral disc, the spinal canal is constricted by the presence of a diffuse annular bulge, anterior buckling of the ligamentum flavum, and shingling of the laminae posteriorly. This

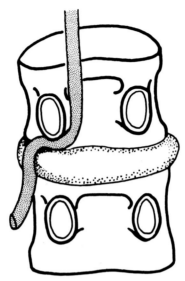

Figure 5.8. In patients suffering from pedicular kinking of the nerve root, it is very common to find at operation that the nerve root is trapped in a gutter formed between a diffuse lateral bulge of the disc and the pedicle above.

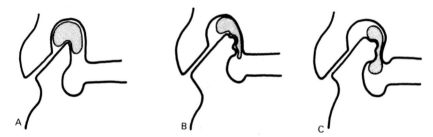

Figure 5.9. The nerve root may be trapped in the foramen. It may be compressed between the tip of a subluxated facet and the pedicle above (*A*), it may be compressed by osteophytic outgrowths on the superior articular facet (*B*), or it may be compressed between the facet and the dorsal aspect of the vertebral body (*C*).

constraint may be further aggravated by overgrowth of the arthritic posterior joints which may indeed also encroach on the midline (Fig. 5.10).

Forward displacement of the laminae seen in degenerative spondylolisthesis and the thickening of the lamina seen in certain pathological states such as fluoridosis and occasionally Paget's disease may produce a posterior encroachment of the spinal canal. Any technqiue of spinal fusion that involves decortication of the laminae with or without the addition of a bone graft may produce a diffuse hypertrophy of the posterior elements leading to constriction of the spinal canal. Postfusion spinal stenosis is, of course, more likely to occur if, prior to surgery, the

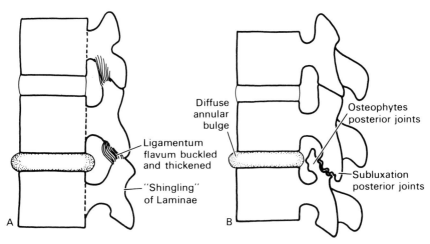

Figure 5.10. In degenerative spinal stenosis, the spinal canal is narrowed by shingling of the laminae and by buckling of the ligamentum flavum. The arthritic posterior joints may hypertrophy and also encroach on the midline giving rise to further compression of the cauda equina. The emerging nerve roots are commonly compressed as they course through the narrow subarticular gutter.

patient was suffering either from a congenital narrowing of the spinal canal or a narrowing produced by degenerative changes of the type previously described. This is most commonly seen at the L4–5 level.

Various combinations and permutations of laminar and apophysial compression are seen. For example, the fifth lumbar nerve root may be compressed as it courses under the superior articular facet at L5, and it may also be trapped in the foramen at the tip of the superior articular facet of S1 (Fig. 5.9). Although laminar compression at times may occur by itself, it is frequently associated with lateral recess or apophysial root entrapment which may arise at the same segment, or the laminar and apophysial compressions may be at different segments (Fig. 5.11).

The Role of HNP in Bony Encroachment

The compression produced in the subarticular gutter by hypertrophy of the posterior facets may be aggravated by a localized protrusion of the annulus and a diffuse annular bulge may critically occlude a segment with a congenital narrowing of the spinal canal. However, although these spatial disc changes augment the degree of compression present, it is important to emphasize the fact that they are not the sole source of compression, and discectomy or chemonucleolysis alone will not relieve the symptoms entirely.

Bony root entrapment, then, results from narrowing of the spinal canal. This narrowing may be apophysial and may compress the nerve roots at their point of emergence at one or more segments. The compression may be in the midline and produced by the lamina, or the root compression may be the result of a combination of both these mechanisms

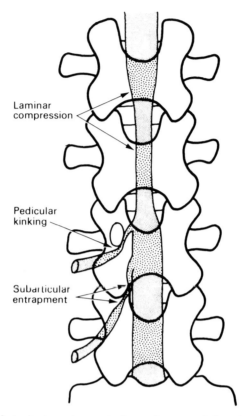

Laminar
compression

Pedicular
kinking

Subarticular
entrapment

Figure 5.11. Spinal stenosis must always be regarded as being laminar and apophysial. Laminar stenosis will compromise the cauda equina: apophysial stenosis will compromise the emerging nerve roots. It is important to recognize, however, as shown in this diagram, that the midline compression may occur at a different level from the apophysial compression of the emerging nerve roots.

at the same level or at different segments. It is important to emphasize that the most common cause of symptoms in spinal stenosis is compression of a nerve root by overgrown facets.

The resulting radicular pain mimics the radicular pain due to a disc rupture. However, the sciatic pain due to a bony root entrapment frequently presents a claudicant character. In contradistinction to the intermittent claudication of vascular insufficiency, the symptoms do not abate on standing still. The patient will give the story that, if the pain strikes him while walking down the road, he will lean forward and rest his hands on his knees to keep his spine in flexion to relieve the symptoms.

CLAUDICANT LEG PAIN

There are several characteristic symptoms which distinguish neurogenic claudication from vascular claudication. Neurogenic claudication is rapid in onset whereas the vascular claudication associated with peripheral vascular disease generally produces symptoms after the patient has walked some distance. The weakness of neurogenic claudication starts proximally and radiates down the leg, whereas vascular claudication (apart from stenosis of the superior gluteal artery) starts in the calf and radiates proximally. With apophysial stenosis, the patient may experience increasing subjective weakness on continuing to walk and may indeed develop objective evidence of impairment of root conduction on re-examination after strenuous activity. Although the peripheral pulses are usually reduced with vascular claudication, if the patient has been sitting for a long time waiting for examination, the pulses may become palpable. In such instances, if there is any suspicion from the history that the patient may be suffering from vascular claudication, then the patient must be examined again after exercise of sufficient severity to bring on the discomfort. Now, on re-examination, it is sometimes impossible to feel the pulses. This is referred to as the "disappearing pulse syndrome."

The claudicant nature of sciatic pain produced by apophysial compression of a nerve root differentiates it from sciatica due to a disc rupture. There are, in addition, several other features that differentiate these two clinical syndromes. The first important difference is the age incidence. Root entrapment by bone is more common over age 50 whereas disc ruptures are more common under age 50. Patients with a bony root entrapment will usually give a history of long-standing backache with

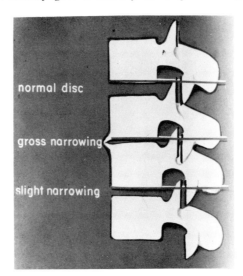

Figure 5.12. When an intervertebral disc narrows, the posterior joints must subluxate. This can be demonstrated on the lateral x-ray by drawing a line along the caudal border of a vertebral body and extending it posteriorly (the joint body line). Normally this line passes over the tip of the superior articular facet. If the posterior joints are subluxated, then this line cuts through the middle of the facet.

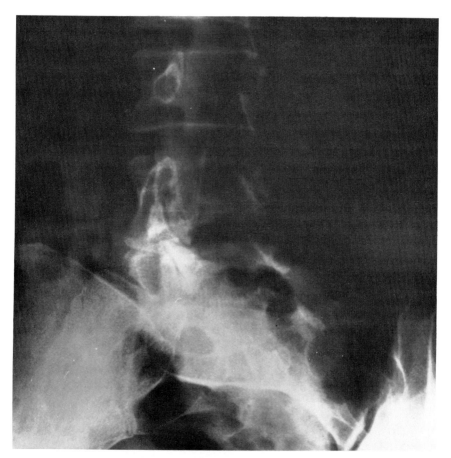

Figure 5.13.   Oblique views showing a crescent-shaped facet joint at L4-5.

the recent gradual onset of sciatica. On examination of a patient with a neurogenic claudication, despite severe sciatic pain, one of the remarkable findings is that straight leg raising is rarely significantly restricted. The bowstring sign and the crossed straight leg raising test are negative. Neurological changes are minimal but, when present, often incriminate more than one root. A true disc rupture with extrusion of nuclear material very rarely occurs at more than one segment simultaneously. This fact is not sufficiently recognized.

A large central disc protrusion, or a protrusion extending laterally into the foramen, or a disc rupture in association with an anomaly of root emergence: though these phenomena may result in the involvement of more than one root, on the whole when there is clinical evidence of multiple root involvement then the probability of bony root entrapment is much greater.

The changes in the intervertebral disc space seen on a routine x-ray of the lumbosacral spine are never of diagnostic significance in a ruptured disc. The demonstration of narrowing of an intervertebral disc does not indict this segment as the site of disc rupture and, indeed in the younger age group, disc protrusions are commonly seen with apparently normal looking discs on routine x-rays.

With apophysial root stenosis, several characteristic changes may be recognized on x-ray. The bony root entrapment syndromes are frequently associated with subluxation of the posterior facets to a marked degree. This can be demonstrated on the lateral view by the fact that the joint body line, a line drawn along the caudal border of the vertebral body,

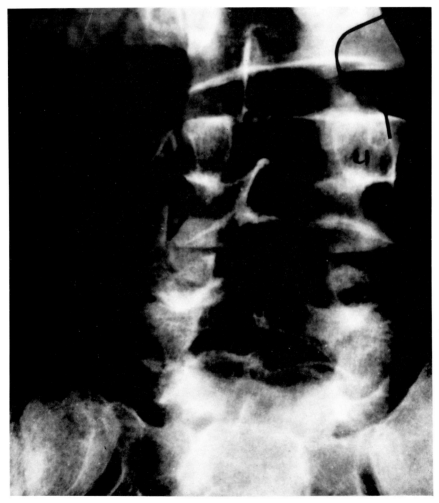

Figure 5.14. In the anteroposterior view, a line drawn along the inferior border of the transverse process over the pars interarticularis and the joint below will form a smooth "S." When subluxation occurs, this line is interrupted. In this x-ray this phenomenon is depicted at the L4-L5 joint on the right.

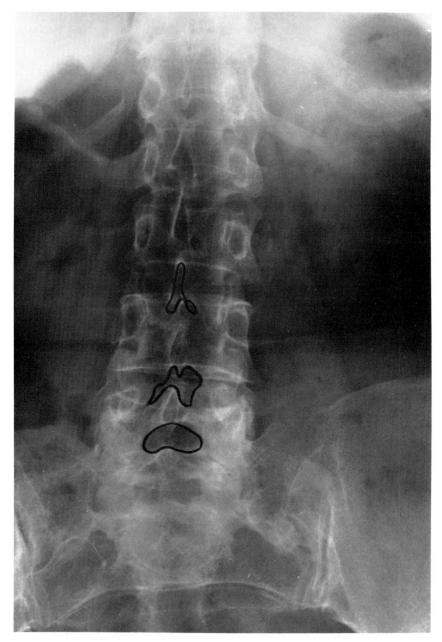

Figure 5.15.   Narrowing of the interlaminar space, most noticeable in outline at the second last and third last mobile levels.

when extended posteriorly, cuts through the middle of the facet instead of passing over the top of it (Fig. 5.12). In chronic subluxations, the inferior articular facet impinges on the lamina below where a reactive ridge of bone is formed. This reactive ridge of bone is recognizable on clinical radiographs as a white crescent on the oblique view (Fig. 5.13).

In the anteroposterior view, a line drawn along the inferior border of the transverse process over the pars interarticularis and the joint below will form a smooth "S." In extreme degrees of subluxation, the tip of the superior articular facet can be seen to impinge against the pedicle above (Fig. 5.14).

Narrowing of the interlaminar space noted in the anteroposterior view of the spine is a very characteristic feature of apophysial stenosis (Fig. 5.15). The interlaminar space may be encroached upon by overgrowth of the posterior facets, by abnormal configuration of the laminae by subluxation of the facets, or by osteoarthritis of the posterior joints.

The findings on myelographic examination differ from those seen with disc ruptures. The myelogram does not show the discreet myelographic defect commonly seen with a rupture of an intervertebral disc (Fig. 5.16). There may be root sleeve cutoff, either unilaterally or bilaterally, and this is best demonstrated by a water-soluble contrast material such as metrizamide. Commonly, on the anteroposterior view, there may be "wasting" of the intrathecal column of water-soluble contrast material (Fig. 5.2A). This myelographic finding is of importance because it may be erroneously interpreted as representing a "central disc rupture."

Degenerative spinal stenosis is frequently associated with a diffuse annular bulge. The posterior hump produced by the diffuse annular bulge as it intrudes into the spinal canal produces a watershed effect (Fig. 5.17). As the dye in the subarachnoid space hurries over this eminence, the increased rate of flow is associated with narrowing of the dye column producing a wasting or hourglass constriction at this segment.

When lateral encroachment is combined with laminar constriction of the spinal canal with or without a diffuse bulge of the annulus, there may be a complete cut-off in the flow of dye (Fig. 5.18). A paintbrush or rat tail appearance at the end of the dye column distinguishes this myelographic defect from that produced by a tumor which shows a characteristic and pathognomonic meniscus (Fig. 5.19).

Laminar compression of the posterior aspects of the cauda equina is revealed on myelography by posterior indentation or even segmentation of the dye column at one or more levels. The fact that the compression is posterior is shown on the lateral view.

In bony root entrapment syndromes, then, the myelograms are difficult to interpret. With increasing sophistication of computerized axial tomography (CAT scanning), it is possible to demonstrate very clearly areas of subarticular narrowing (Fig. 5.20). However, there may be narrowing at several segments, and the mere presence of this change, therefore, does

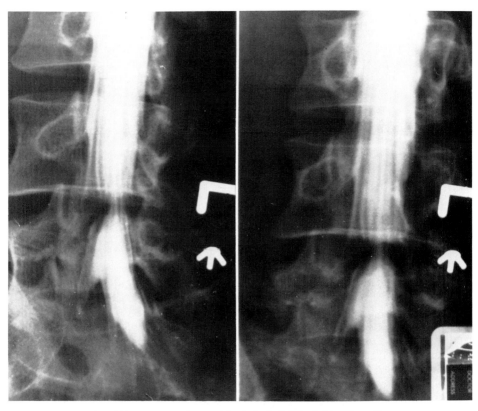

Figure 5.16. Discreet myelographic defect, L4-5 right. Note first root inter-ference from L4-5 HNP.

not necessarily mean the nerve root is compromised at this level. In such instances, therefore, it is frequently necessary to determine the level of root involvement by root sleeve infiltration and by electromyography (*cf.* Chapter 9).

The source of the leg pain, in these patients, is compression of an emerging nerve root by bony overgrowth and in such instance, even if this compression is augmented by a localized annular bulge, it is impossible to give relief of symptoms by the intradiscal injection of chymopapain.

Chemonucleolysis is indicated solely for the extradural compression of a nerve root by a ruptured intervertebral disc. It has no place in other forms of root entrapment.

Finally, consideration must be given to a strong ligamentous band that runs from the transverse process to the vertebral body. Although this is not described in standard books on anatomy, it was a constant finding in our dissections and we call it the corporo-transverse ligament (Fig. 5.21).

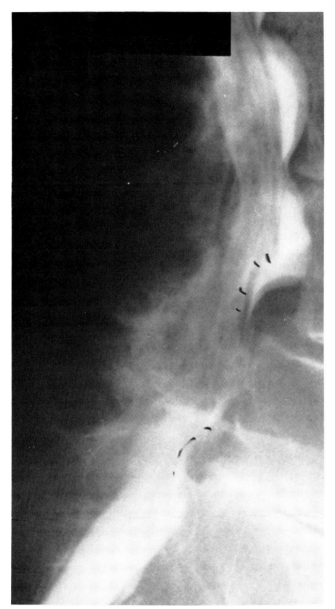

Figure 5.17. Watershed effect by multiple anterior defects.

At the lumbosacral level, the fifth root courses between this ligament and the ala of the sacrum. With disc collapse, the edge of the ligament descends on the nerve root and may trap it against the ala of the sacrum. The clinical picture is indistinguishable from bony root entrapment.

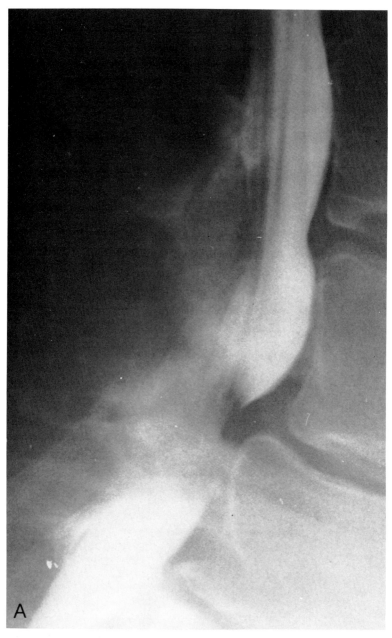

Figure 5.18.   Complete block on myelography (with slight rat-tail appearance) occurring at a level of degenerative spondylolisthesis.

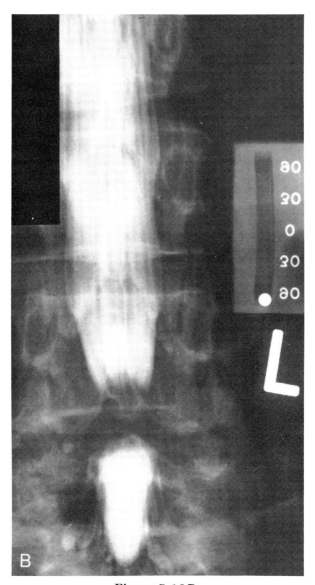

Figure 5.18*B*.

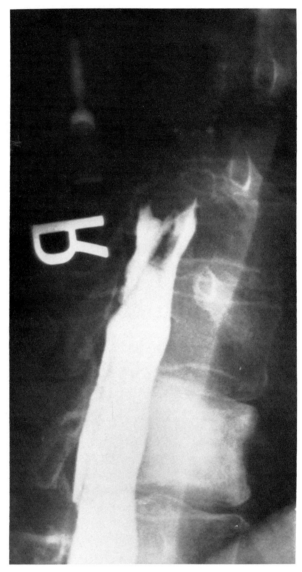

Figure 5.19.   Myelogram showing intradural tumor meniscus.

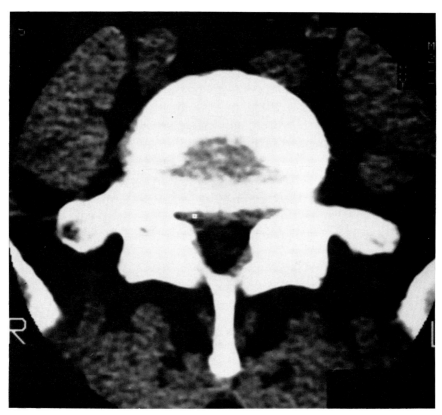

Figure 5.20. CT scan showing lateral recess stenosis with diffuse disc bulge.

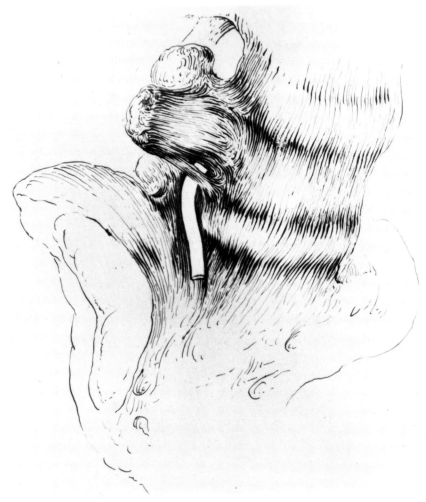

Figure 5.21.   The relationship of the fifth lumbar nerve root to the corporo-transverse ligament.

   Chemonucleolysis is only useful for the patient with sciatica due to an HNP. Symptoms arising out of bony encroachment on nerve roots will not resolve with the intradiscal injection of any proteolytic enzyme.
   An HNP is not just a defect on myelography or CT scan.
   An HNP is not just a story of pain down the leg.
   An HNP causing sciatica is a combination of historical features, physical findings, and supportive myelographic or CT examination described in Chapter 6.

References

1. Sinclair DC, Feindel WH, Waddell G, *et al.*: The intervertebral ligaments as a source of segmental pain. *J Bone Joint Surg* 308:515, 1948.
2. Mixter WJ, Barr JS: Rupture of the intervertebral disc with involvement of the spinal canal. *N Engl J Med* 211:210, 1934.
3. Dandy WE: Concealed ruptured intervertebral disks. *JAMA* 117:821, 1941.
4. American Academy of Orthopaedic Surgeons: *A Glossary on Spinal Terminology.* 1981.
5. Falconer MA, McGeorge M, Begg CA: Observations on the cause and mechanism of symptom-production in sciatica and low-back pain. *J Neurol Neurosurg Psychiatry* 11:13, 1948.
6. McCulloch JA: *Computed Tomography Before and After Chemonucleolysis* (in print).
7. Howe JF: *A Neurophysiological Basis for the Radicular Pain of Nerve Root Compression:* Advances in Pain Research and Therapy, Vol. 3. New York, Raven Press, 1979.
8. Verbiest H: A radicular syndrome from developmental narrowing of the lumbar vertebral canal. *J Bone Joint Surg* 36:230, 1954.
9. Schatzker J, Pennal GF: Spinal stenosis, a cause of cauda equina compression. *J Bone Joint Surg* 50:606, 1968.

CHAPTER 6

The Clinical Syndrome of Lumbar Root Compression Due to Disc Rupture

The authors make no excuse for repeating the fact that chemonucle-olysis is only of value in the treatment of patients in whom the symptom of sciatic pain is due to compromise of lumbar nerve root by rupture of an intervertebral disc. A disc rupture, although varied in its presentation, tends to have a fairly consistent group of symptoms and signs. The common 'o garden type of disc herniation will be described in this chapter and the subtle variations will be covered in more detail in Chapter 9.

CLINICAL PICTURE
History

Approximately half of the patients will attribute their attack to various forms of traumatic experience. This is retrograde rationalization on the part of the patient. Experimental studies and careful statistical analysis of case histories do not support the concept that direct trauma or sudden weight-loading of the spine are the causal agents of disc rupture, although they may aggravate a pre-existing lesion. This aspect in the history becomes important when litigation or compensation is involved.

In a few patients, especially younger ones, sciatica is the only symptom. If asked specifically, many patients may volunteer the information that the first symptom noted before the pain developed was numbness in the calf or foot. This is a stage of root compression before the inflammatory radiculitis begins. The majority of patients, however, develop back pain which subsequently radiates to the buttock and then down the leg. Most patients report that, as the sciatic pain increases, the back pain decreases in severity. The history of pain is spondylogenic in character. That is to say, the pain is aggravated by general and specific activities and is relieved by rest. Bending, stooping, lifting, coughing, sneezing, and straining at stool will intensify the pain. The complaint of an increase in pain in the involved extremity after sitting for a period of time, particularly on a toilet seat, is of great diagnostic significance. Infrequently unusual referral patterns of pain occur such as perineal or testicular discomfort (pain or paresthesia) and lower abdominal discomfort. The former symptoms are likely due to irritation of lower sacral roots laterally or midline and the latter may be due to muscular splinting of the pelvis.

It is unreliable to attempt to identify the root involved by asking the patient to describe the anatomical distribution of the pain in the leg. However, in general, pain derived from the L5 and S1 roots courses down the posterior aspect of the leg, whereas lesions of the third and fourth lumbar roots give rise to pain on the anterior part of the thigh. It is routine for sciatic pain, due to fifth and first root compression, to radiate below the knee. But you will occasionally see a younger patient with pain off to one iliac crest region or just into the buttock, who, with investigation, has herniated nucleus pulposus (HNP). It is safe to teach that all sciatic pain due to root compression radiates below the knee, but there are exceptions to every generalization in medicine.

Paresthesia in the form of tingling, numbness, or a sensation of something trickling down the leg are common and may be of value in localizing the level of root compression. It is interesting to note that, although pain is more marked proximally (in the buttocks and upper thigh), numbness and tingling are more common in the leg and foot.

Rarely the only leg symptom may be numbness in the foot and in the lower leg. The numbness is often vaguely localized and may have a stocking-like distribution suggestive of a neuropathy or a psychogenic regional pain syndrome. Rarely, motor symptoms predominate and are more disabling than the pain. In such instances, the clinician has to beware of the presence of a spinal tumor or peripheral neuropathy.

Physical Examination

THE BACK

The posture is characteristic. The lumbar spine is flattened and slightly flexed. The patient often leans away from the side of his pain and this sciatic scoliosis becomes more obvious if he tries to bend forward. The patient is more comfortable if he stands with the affected hip and knee slightly flexed, a manner accentuated by asking the patient to flex forward (Fig. 6.1). He walks in obvious discomfort, frequently holding his loin with his hands. His gait is slow and deliberate and is designed to avoid any unnecessary movement of his spine. With gross tension on the nerve root, the patient may not be able to put his heel on the ground and walks slowly and painfully on tiptoe.

Forward flexion may be permitted so the hands reach the knees by virtue of flexion of the hip joint. If the examiner keeps his fingertips on the spinous processes, he can see that the lumbar spine hardly moves at all. Limitation of flexion in such instances is, therefore, the result of root tension. The degree of flexion should be recorded by measuring the distance between the fingertips and the floor.

Extension is also limited, although to a lesser degree than flexion, and in most instances the pelvis starts to rotate as soon as the patient attempts to lean backwards. The complaint on extension is usually back pain but at times the patient may feel leg pain.

Lateral flexion may be full and free but, in the presence of a sciatic scoliosis, lateral flexion towards the convexity of the curve (side of sciatica) is limited.

The phenomenon of sciatic scoliosis and the relief or aggravation of pain on lateral flexion have been attributed to the position of the protrusion in relation to the nerve root (Fig. 6.2). However, this may be a simplistic explanation in view of the fact that the sciatic scoliosis disappears on recumbency. This observation, the loss of lateral curvature of the lumbar spine on recumbency, differentiates the sciatic list from a structural scoliosis. On further assessment of the degree of root involvement present, it is imperative to test specifically for root tension, root irritation, and impairment of root conduction. These are the cardinal signs of lumbar root compromise.

TENDERNESS AND MUSCLE SPASM

In the standing position, especially in the presence of scoliosis, muscle spasm can be observed. However at rest, the spasm often subsides and there is little tenderness to be found on examination. Selectively palpat-

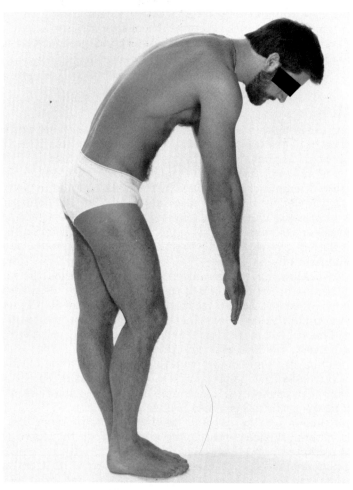

Figure 6.1. Typical posture on flexion with nerve root tension causing knee flexion and pelvic rotation.

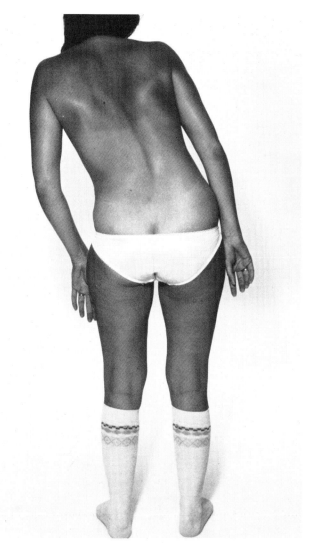

Figure 6.2.   Sciatic scoliosis, tilt to the left. The patient had an HNP, L5-S1 right.

ing and applying a lateral thrust to the spinous process may cause some back pain and on rare occasions produce leg pain. By and large, in the patient with sciatica due to an HNP, at complete rest in the prone position on the examining table, there is little to find in the back. The patient's major complaint is leg pain and the majority of physical findings are in the extremities.

THE EXTREMITIES

Root Tension and Irritation

The term, "root tension," denotes distortion of the emerging nerve root by an extradural lesion. The two most useful tests for the presence of root tension are limitation of straight leg raising and the bowstring sign, the latter also arising in part from root irritation.

When testing straight leg raising, it is important not to hurt the patient. Never jerk the leg up in the air suddenly. The knee must be kept fully extended by firm pressure exerted by the examiner's hand and the hip internally rotated and adducted slightly. With the other hand under the heel, the examiner *slowly* raises the leg until leg pain or back pain is produced (Fig. 6.3).

Two additional maneuvers are of vital importance to add significance to the finding of limitation of straight leg raising:
1. Aggravation of pain by forced dorsiflexion of the ankle at the limit of straight leg raising.
2. Relief of pain by flexion of the knee and hip.

Physiogenic sciatic pain due to nerve root compromise is always relieved by flexion of the knee and hip. Further flexion of the patient's

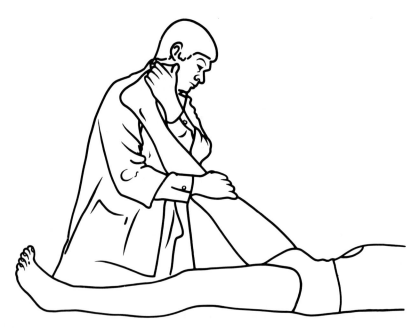

Figure 6.3. When carrying out the straight leg raising test, it is important to remember that the leg should be raised *slowly* and during this movement, the knee must be maintained in the fully extended position by the examiner's hand.

hip with the knee bent does not reproduce and aggravate sciatic pain. This phenomenon is only seen in the emotionally destroyed.

If straight leg raising is permissible to 70° before leg pain is produced, the finding is equivocal for an HNP. Below this level the reproduction of leg pain on straight leg raising, aggravated by dorsiflexion of the ankle and relieved by flexion of the knee, is strongly suggestive of tension on the fifth lumbar or first sacral roots. Reproduction of the sciatic pain in the affected extremity by raising the unaffected leg is irrefutable evidence of root tension (contralateral or crossed straight leg raising).

In patients in whom numbness in the foot is a predominant symptom, repetitive straight leg raising, i.e., "pumping of the leg," frequently intensifies the sensation of numbness.

Location of Pain on Straight Leg Raising

The examiner is seeking to reproduce leg (buttock, thigh, and calf) pain when doing the straight leg raising (SLR) test. Reproduction of back pain, especially in the high ranges of SLR testing is usually not indicative of root tension. However, there is one exception which is discussed under midline disc herniation in Chapter 9.

False Positive Straight Leg Raising Test

Hamstring tightness may cloud the assessment of the SLR test. Remember that these patients have a generally tight body build (e.g., inability to fully extend the elbow) and miles of room between the wrist flexed, thumb abducted position and the volar surface of the forearm (Fig. 6.4, A and B). Hamstring tightness should be bilateral and the discomfort the patient witnesses is distal in the thigh in the region of the hamstring tendons. Hamstring tightness does not produce pain radiating below the knee. Finally, other physical findings of root tension, irritation, and compression are absent in hamstring tightness.

False Negative Straight Leg Raising Test

On occasion you will encounter a loose jointed individual with sciatica due to an HNP. On SLR testing you may not be impressed with the degree of impaired SLR until you examine the unaffected leg and see the patient's ability to straight leg raise well beyond 90°.

The Bowstring Sign

The bowstring sign is an important indication of root tension and irritation. The examiner carries out straight leg raising to the point at which the patient experiences some discomfort in the distribution of the sciatic nerve. At this level, the knee is allowed to flex and the patient's foot is allowed to rest on the examiner's shoulder (Fig. 6.5). The test demands sudden, firm pressure applied to the popliteal nerve in the popliteal fossa. The action may startle the patient enough to make him jump, and this jump may hurt. To prevent this, first of all, tell the patient that you are just going to press firmly on the back of the knee. Apply firm pressure to the hamstrings: this will not hurt. Then, move your

thumbs over to the popliteal nerve. Apply sudden, firm pressure with
your thumb over the popliteal nerve. A positive bowstring test is reproduction of radiating leg discomfort. Most commonly the radiating discomfort is pain felt proximally in the thigh and even into the back. Less

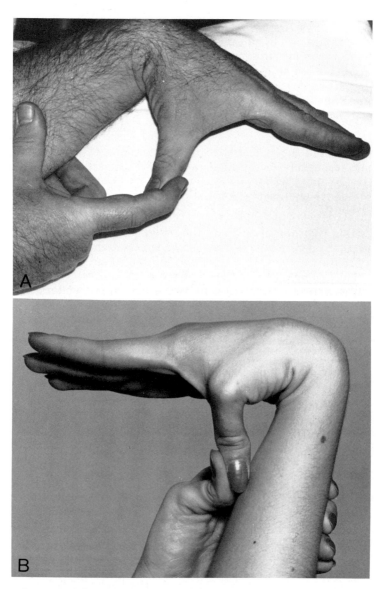

Figure 6.4. *A*, tight-jointed individual. Thumb cannot be made to touch volar
surface of forearm. *B*, loose-jointed individual. Thumb easily touches forearm.

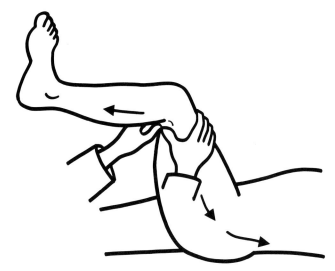

Figure 6.5. When eliciting the bowstring sign the patient's foot should be allowed to rest on the examiner's shoulder with the knee very slightly flexed at the limit of straight leg raising. Sudden firm pressure is then applied to the examiner's thumbs in the popliteal fossa. Radiation of pain down the leg or the production of pain in the back is pathognomonic of root tension.

commonly radiating discomfort will travel distally and this discomfort is more often paresthetic in nature than painful. It is important to emphasize that, if the test only produces local pain in the popliteal fossa, then it is of no significance. This demonstration of root irritation is probably the single most important sign in the diagnosis of tension and irritation of a nerve root by a ruptured intervertebral disc.

Tests to Verify SLR Reduction

When the patient sits with the knees dangling over the side of the bed, the hip and knee are both flexed to 90°. If the knee is now extended fully, the position assumed by the leg is equivalent to 90° of straight leg raising (Fig. 6.6). If the patient is suffering from root compromise, this will cause sudden, severe pain and the patient will throw his trunk backwards to avoid tension on the nerve. This is commonly referred to as the "positive flip test." With the psychogenic regional pain syndrome, the patient will permit the examiner to extend the knee of the painful leg without showing any response at all.

If the patient complains of severe sciatic pain when attempting to bend forwards and there is a suspicion that there may be a significant degree of functional overlay, the patient should be asked to kneel on a chair. This will relax the hamstrings and the sciatic nerve. With the patient kneeling on the chair, he is now asked to bend forward. With a physiogenic source of pain, then the patient will be able to bend the spine and let his fingertips go below the level of the seat. In the psychogenic regional pain phenomenon, even with the knee flexed and the patient kneeling on a chair, he will not allow the spine to bend (Fig. 6.7).

Nerve root pain is probably the result of a combination of pressure and an inflammatory response to the prolapsed disc material. This "inflammatory response," this "radiculitis" has been loosely termed "root irritation." Root irritation is an important factor in the demonstrated limitation of straight leg raising and it would appear to be productive of peripheral muscle tenderness. Such tenderness is not always present but, if demonstrable, it is of value in localizing the level of root involvement. Frequently the calf is tender with S1 lesions, the anterior tibial compartment with L5 root involvement, and the quadriceps is tender when the fourth lumbar nerve root has been compromised.

The shin is the body image of the leg and very marked tenderness on palpating the subcutaneous surface of the tibia should warn the clinician that the patient has a large emotional content in his total disability. In the psychogenic regional pain syndromes (Chapter 8), the patient frequently has skin tenderness with pain on just pinching the skin. Obviously, no meaningful statement can be made of the presence of deep muscle tenderness unless skin tenderness has been tested first. This is a trap for the unwary.

It should be noted that the upper outer quadrant of the buttock is a

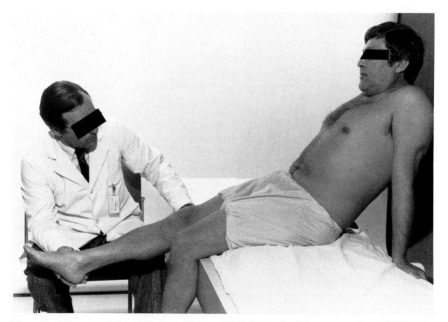

Figure 6.6. Positive flip test. When SLR is limited because of an HNP, the patient flips backwards to relieve nerve root tension.

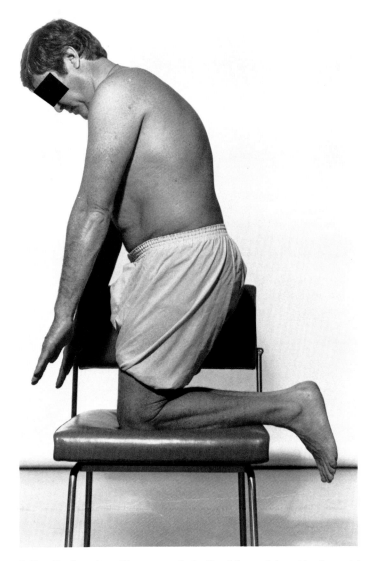

Figure 6.7. Patient kneeling on a chair. In this position, the hamstrings are relaxed, and the tension on the sciatic nerve is reduced. Reluctance to flex the spine while in this position is indictive of a psychogenic pain phenomenon.

tender area in most people, with or without backache, and this area becomes increasingly tender in the presence of root irritation at any segment. The demonstration of this tenderness is of no localizing value. Patients with discogenic back pain with root irritation may also have tenderness over the sacroiliac joints and down the course of the sciatic nerve. This referred tenderness over the sacroiliac joint has given rise to confusion in the past resulting in the diagnosis of "sacroiliac strain" without any other clinical evidence or radiological evidence of damage to the sacroiliac joint.

Femoral Nerve Stretch-

Figure 6.8 shows the femoral nerve stretch test. It is not nearly as satisfactory a test as SLR, but it is positive when unilateral thigh pain is produced and aggravated by knee flexion. It is difficult to interpret in the presence of hip pathology.

Impairment of Root Conduction

The diagnosis of disc rupture is in no way exclusively dependent on the demonstration of root impairment as reflected by signs of motor weakness or changes in sensory appreciation or reflex activity. However, the presence of such changes reinforces the diagnosis.

Changes in Reflex Activity. The ankle jerk may be diminished or absent with an S1 lesion. This is tested with the patient kneeling on a chair or sitting comfortably. (If a patient's sciatica is so bad he cannot sit with comfort, then do not test any reflex in the sitting position as the guarding and posturing the patient will do to try to become more comfortable will upset the assessment of reflexes. This explains the occasional depression of a knee reflex seen in the presence of sciatica

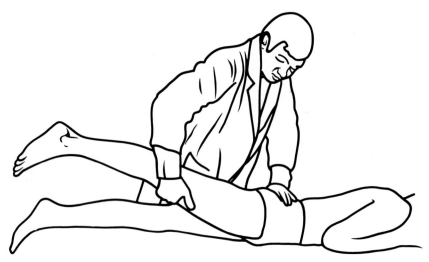

Figure 6.8. When the fourth lumbar nerve is compromised, the patient experiences pain radiating down the front of the thigh. This pain will be aggravated if the hip is extended with the knees slightly flexed. It is to be noted that this test may give rise to back pain by virtue of hyperextending the spine, but this finding is not of diagnostic significance.

due to an L5-S1 disc protrusion.) If the patient has suffered from a previous attack of sciatic pain with significant compression of the first sacral nerve to obliterate the ankle jerk, this may not return to normal. The absence of ankle jerk, therefore, may merely be a stigma of a previous episode of disc rupture and the present attack may be due to a disc rupture at another level. Scratching the sole of the foot, as in the plantar response, produces a reflex contraction of the tensor fascia femoris. This little known reflex is often lost with an S1 lesion.

With an L5 root compression, the tibialis posterior reflex obtained by striking the tendon of the tibialis posterior near its point of insertion may be absent. This is a pure L5 response. The clinician has to practice obtaining this reflex; it is not easy to elicit. Diminution of the hamstring jerk is also seen on occasion with an L5 root compromise, but multiple innervation of this muscle group makes this an unreliable reflex.

With L4 and L3 lesions, the knee jerk may be diminished. Many other deep tendon reflexes can be tested; however, assessment of the reflexes mentioned above has been of the greatest value in the routine assessment of the clinical syndrome of the ruptured disc.

The common neurological changes are summarized in Table 6.1.

Wasting. Muscle wasting is rarely seen unless the symptoms have been present for more than 3 weeks. Very marked wasting is more suggestive of an extradural tumor than of a disc rupture.

The girth of the thigh and the girth of the calf should always be measured. This will act as a base line, on occasion, to assess the progress of the lesion. It must be remembered that, if there is gross weakness of the gastrocnemii, the main venous pump of the affected extremity is no longer working and these patients may indeed show some measure of ankle edema. The combination of calf tenderness due to S1 root irritation and the observation of a swollen ankle may give rise to the erroneous diagnosis of a thrombophlebitis.

Motor Loss. The weakness of the gastrocnemii is best demonstrated by getting the patient to rise on tiptoe five or six times. The patient is

Table 6.1.
Common Neurological Changes in HNP

Change	Root		
	L4	L5	S1
Motor weakness	Knee extension	Ankle dorsiflexion	Ankle plantar flexion
Sensory loss	Medial shin to knee	Dorsum of foot and lateral calf	Lateral border of foot and posterior calf
Reflex depression	Knee	Tibialis posterior	Ankle
Wasting	Thigh (no calf)	Calf (minimal thigh)	Calf (minimal thigh)

asked if it requires more effort to rise on tiptoe on the affected extremity. If the quadriceps is weak, the physician must be wary of this before ascribing the difficulty of tiptoe rising to weakness of the calf muscles or, if sciatic pain is severe, the test cannot be performed by the patient. Jumping on tiptoe may be painful and it is not a good method of examination although slight weakness may be assessed by asking the patient to walk backwards and forwards across the length of the examining room on tiptoes to find out whether the gastrocnemii tire more easily.

The power of ankle dorsiflexion is best tested by applying full body weight to the dorsiflexed ankle (Fig. 6.9). Testing the dorsiflexors by asking the patient to walk on his heels will only demonstrate marked weakness in this muscle group. Weakness of the flexor hallucis longus (S1) or weakness of the extensor hallucis longus (L5) is often the first evidence of motor involvement. The evertors of the foot may be weak with an L5 lesion. The gluteus maximus may become weak with lesions involving the first sacral nerve root and may be demonstrated by the sagging of one buttock crease when the patient stands. Weakness of the gluteus medius is seen with an L5 lesion and occasionally is marked enough to produce a Trendelenberg lurch, particularly noticeable when the patient is tired. When the gluteus medius is involved, there is frequently marked tenderness on pressure over the muscle near its point

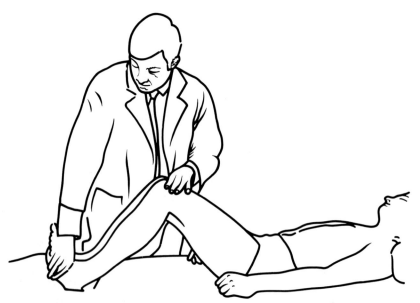

Figure 6.9. The power of the dorsiflexors of the ankle should be tested with the patient lying on his back with his hips and knees flexed. The patient holds his ankle in full dorsiflexion and attempts to resist the maximal force that the physician can apply to the dorsum of the foot.

of insertion and this may be confused with a trochanteric bursitis or with gluteal tendonitis.

Quadriceps weakness is seen with an L4 lesion and can be assessed by the examiner placing his arm under the patient's knee and asking the patient to extend the knee against the resistance of the examiner's hand. However, this maneuver may produce pain and a false impression of weakness is obtained. In such instances, it is better to have the patient lying face downwards and flexing his knees to 90° and then assessing the power to fully extend the knee from this position (Fig. 6.10).

Sensory Impairment. The regions of sensory loss are reasonably constant. There appear to be areas more vulnerable to sensory loss than others. Loss of appreciation of pinprick is first noted in an S1 lesion below and behind the lateral malleolus and in an L5 lesion in the cleft between the first and second toes. Sensory appreciation is a subjective response and, as such, may at times be difficult to assess. Certain precautions must be followed. Sensory sensibility varies in different parts of the limb. Identical areas in each limb must be tested consecutively. The examination must be carried out as expeditiously as compatible with accuracy because the patient will soon tire of this form of examination and his answers may not be accurate. When the skin is pricked with a pin, the physiological principle of recruitment is present. The overall sensory appreciation is dependent, then, not only on the action of the pinprick, but also on the number of pinpricks experienced.

A sensory examination is only interpreted as positive when the sensory

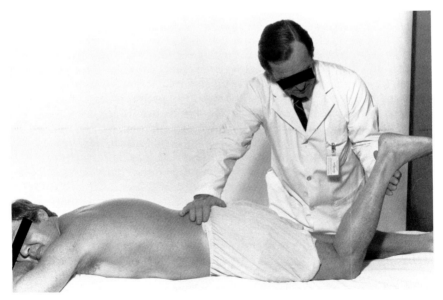

Figure 6.10.   The most comfortable position for testing quadriceps weakness.

loss approximates one dermatomal distribution, and the loss is not present in the adjacent dermatomes or the same contralateral dermatome.

Patients over the age of 50 frequently demonstrate a delay in evaluating a sensory stimulus applied to the lower extremity. This is particularly applicable to the differentiation between hot and cold.

RADIOGRAPHIC EXAMINATION

The major value of x-rays of the lumbar spine in the routine assessment of a disc rupture is to exclude more serious pathology, such as tumors or infections that may mimic the syndrome. X-rays are not of localizing value. The demonstration of a narrowed disc space does not necessarily indicate that this represents the involved segment.

Myelography, however, should only be employed if the surgeon has decided that the disability experienced by the patient, despite adequate conservative treatment, had reached a stage where consideration must be given, either to laminectomy or to chemonucleolysis. Myelography has three purposes: firstly, to localize the exact level of root involvement and secondly, to exclude the presence of a sequestrated disc that has migrated proximally or distally and is, therefore, not susceptible to treatment by intradiscal injection of chymopapain (Fig. 6.11). The fragment is no longer attached physically to the disc from which it extruded. Thirdly, myelography helps rule out unusual pathology such as tumors.

It is not the purpose of this text to discuss in detail the radiological changes that may be seen on myelography but some general principles regarding interpretation of myelograms are described.

Myelography was introduced in 1921 by Sicard (2) using iodized poppyseed oil injected into the epidural space. This is a logical place to put radiopaque material because the lesion is, indeed, an epidural lesion and should be demonstrated more easily by a radiopaque substance introduced into the epidural space. However, difficulty in aspirating the radiopaque material at the conclusion of the epidural myelography and the suggestion that this might give rise to root irritation at a later date persuaded surgeons to use the intrathecal injection of oil-soluble radiopaque compounds. Because these compounds are immulsified with the cerebrospinal fluid, it is not possible in the majority of instances to aspirate all of the dye injected.

Over the past several years, an impression has been gleaned that myelography is not a totally innocuous procedure. Apart from the discomforts attendant upon myelography, there has been a suggestion that the oil-soluble dye acts as an irritant and may in its early postexamination phase be the initiating agent in transverse myelitis (3) and in the later stages be the initiating agent for a progressive arachnoiditis (4).

Water-soluble opaque material would appear preferable in that it is totally absorbed and does not leave any residual irritating radiopaque material in the subarachnoid space.

The original water-soluble compounds proved to be a little hazardous and were frequently associated with the production of epileptiform seizures (3). Metrizamide, however, has proven to be relatively innocuous although the patients may have unpleasant side effects if the dye is run up the neck and is allowed to spill over into the cranium.

The metrizamide routine is as follows:

1. The patient is allowed to eat and drink before the procedure.
2. The patient is encouraged to drink extra fluids before and after the procedure.
3. The study is confined to the lowest thoracic and all lumbar levels.
4. The patient is kept in the semirecumbant position for 4 to 6 hours post injection.
5. Barbiturates (phenobarbital, 60 mg PO × 2) are given to prevent convulsions.
6. Phenothiazines and related drugs should be avoided.

Metrizamide has several advantages over oil-soluble myelography in that it flows more easily, it can be injected with a smaller needle, and the dye will flow down the root sleeve into the root canal. It gives a more sensitive demonstration of an extradural or extraradicular lesion.

With oil-soluble myelography, a significant disc rupture may be present without producing any myelographic defect under the following circumstances. If the lesion is very lateral, it will not encroach on the dural sac and will not create a flow defect. Similarly, defects may not be seen if the dural sac is narrow or if it does not extend caudally to the sacrum (Fig. 6.12, A and B). The dural sac tapers as it approaches the sacrum and, for these reasons, a falsely negative myelogram is most commonly seen at the lumbosacral junction if an oil-soluble contrast material is employed. With water-soluble contrast material filling the nerve root adequately, a lumbosacral disc rupture will be demonstrated by lack of filling of the first sacral root (Fig. 6.12, C and D).

A diffuse bulge of the annulus arising as a result of disc degeneration is most commonly encountered at L4-5. The posterior hump, as it intrudes into the spinal canal, produces a watershed effect. As the dye in the subarachnoid space hurries over this eminence, the increased rate of flow is associated with a narrowing of the dye column, producing wasting or hourglass constriction at this segment (Fig. 5.2A). This x-ray appearance is frequently erroneously referred to as a central disc. Very frequently with a degenerative spinal stenosis, it can be seen that the indentation in the oil column is made more obvious by hypertrophy of the posterior facets which intrude towards the midline. It is to be noted that radicular symptoms associated with this type of disc lesion are usually due to the assciated spinal stenosis. Because of the concomitant bony root entrapment, chemonucleolysis is unlikely to be of any value whatsoever.

In general, it can be said that false negative myelograms are more commonly seen at the L5-S1 level and false positive myelograms are more commonly noted at the L4-5 level.

EPIDURAL VENOGRAPHY

The epidural veins are remarkably constant in their anatomical disposition (Fig. 6.13). The anterior internal vertebral veins run vertically and lie in close apposition to the intervertebral discs. A laterally placed

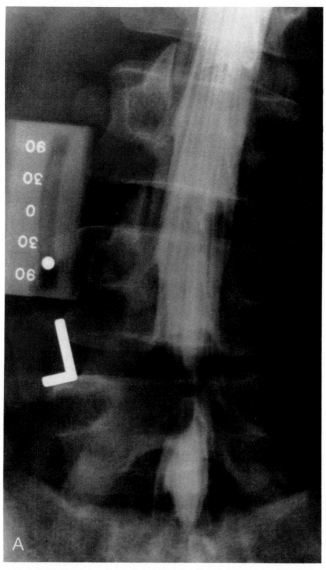

Figure 6.11. *A* and *B*, metrizamide myelogram (radiculogram) showing most of the contrast column defect behind the body of L5, indicating a probable sequestered disc.

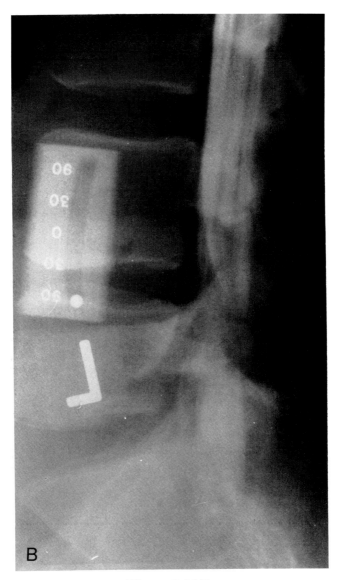

Figure 6.11*B*.

disc rupture not demonstrable on myelography in a patient with a short or narrow dural sac can be demonstrated by the fact that the flow in the vertebral vein running over the disc protrusion is interrupted. The vertebral veins lying with the spinal canal communicate by the radicular veins with longitudinal venous channels immediately anterior to the

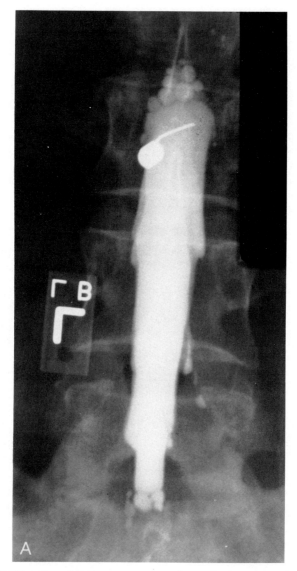

Figure 6.12. *A* and *B*, Pantopaque myelography interpreted as normal.

transverse processes. These radicular veins run in close apposition to the
nerve roots as they course through the intervertebral foramina.

The epidural veins can be outlined by the percutaneous catheterization
of the femoral vein and advancement of the catheter into the external
vertebral vein under x-ray control. With the vertebral venous plexus
clearly outlined by the injection of contrast material, interruption of the
venous flow can be readily demonstrated (Fig. 6.14).

ELECTROMYOGRAPHY

Evaluation of the electrical activities of muscles, either at rest or with contraction, may be used to localize the level of lumbar nerve root involvement. Healthy, normally innervated muscle is electrically "silent" at rest and the insertion of an electromyographic needle does not produce sustained electrical discharges. However, in the presence of a root lesion, a series of involuntary electrical discharges can be recorded. These are characterized by a shortened potential and reduced amplitude (*fibrillation potentials*) or by altered wave forms (*positive waves*). The positive wave forms are only produced on needle insertion, but the fibrillation potentials can be recorded all the time.

On voluntary contraction of a normal muscle, the action potentials evoke a biphasic or triphasic form. With partial denervation, the quantity

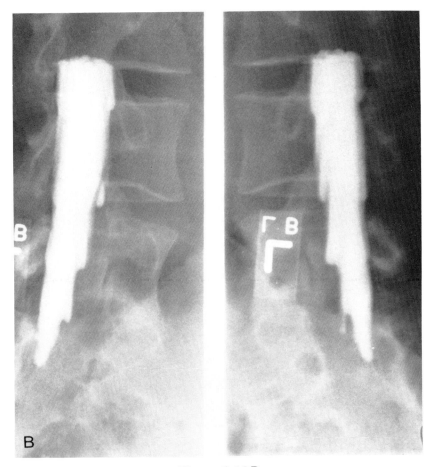

Figure 6.12*B*.

of motor units recorded is decreased and multiple polyphasic waves are seen (Fig. 6.15).

The paraspinal muscles are supplied by the posterior primary rami of the emerging lumbar nerve roots. In the electromyographic examination of a patient suffering from nerve root compression, the electrical activity

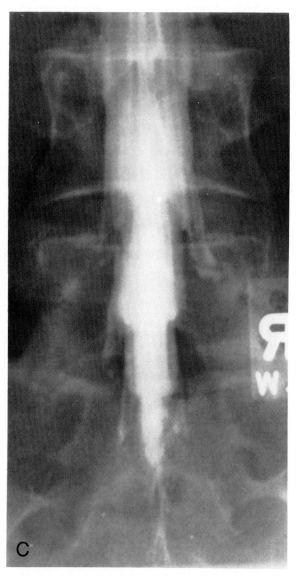

Figure 6.12.   *C* and *D*, metrizamide myelography done 3 months later when symptoms persisted. It shows root cut-off, L5-S1 right.

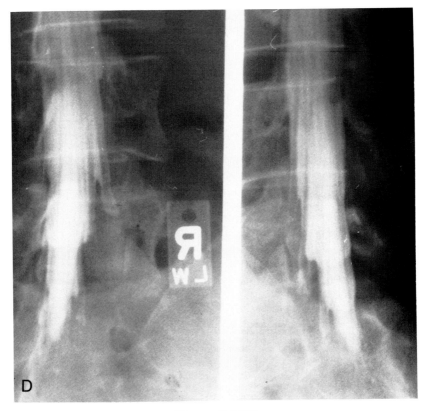

Figure 6.12D.

of the paraspinal muscles at rest and on voluntary activity must be recorded.

It is to be noted that operative exposure of the lumbar spine invariably damages the posterior primary rami. After surgery, paraspinal electromyography reveals partial denervation or abnormal electrical potentials. In a series we studied, these changes were found to persist for as long as 15 years. Paraspinal electromyography is, therefore, of little or no diagnostic value in assessing the level of root involvement in a patient who has undergone previous spinal surgery.

There is a regrettable tendency when reporting the diagnostic accuracy of electromyography and myelography to compare the two. They are not, however, alternative methods of examination; they should be used to supplement each other. Electromyography is able to localize specific root involvement but does not give any information as to the site or nature of the lesion. Myelography, on the other hand, gives information in regard to the anatomical location of the lesion and the probable pathology.

Theoretically, because of the short distance between the muscles supplied and the root itself, changes in the paraspinal muscles detected by electromyography should be more accurate in localizing the level of root involvement and changes in the peripheral muscles.

In an S1 lesion, the examination can be broadened to include the sensory limb of the sciatic nerve. It is possible to stimulate the afferent limb of S1 with an electrode in the popliteal fossa and to measure the time required to travel to the dorsal root, pass through the reflex arc, travel down the efferent limb, and eventually produce a contraction of the gastrocnemius. This is the Hoffmann reflex, sometimes referred to as the H-reflex. With S1 root involvement, the time between the sensory stimulus and the motor response will be prolonged, and the pattern of the evoked potential may be abnormal. However, it must be remembered that, if the patient does not have an ankle jerk, the Hoffmann reflex will be abnormal. The Hoffmann reflex, therefore, is of diagnostic value only in those patients who clinically appear to have an S1 lesion and in whom the ankle jerk is still maintained.

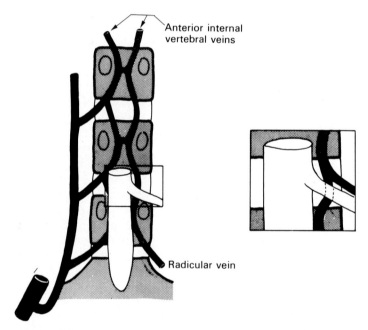

Anterior internal vertebral veins

Radicular vein

Figure 6.13. Diagram to show the disposition of the anterior internal vertebral veins and the radicular veins. It can be seen that the anterior internal vertebral veins are closely apposed to the intervertebral disc and that the radicular veins cross the intervertebral disc accompanying the nerve roots as they emerge through the intervertebral foramina.

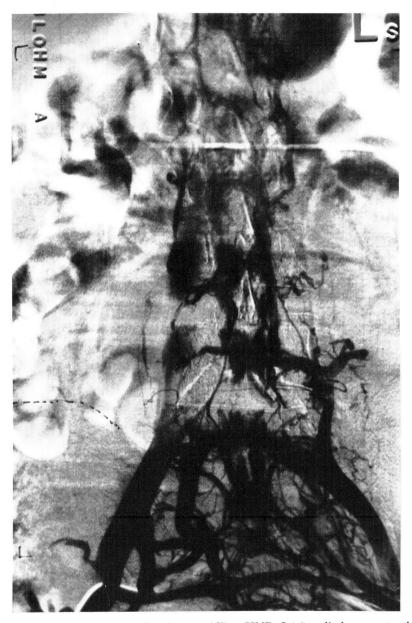

Figure 6.14. Venogram showing a midline HNP, L4-5, a little more to the right than left side.

DISCOGRAPHY

When the technique of discography was originally introduced, it was hoped that the demonstration of posterior extravasation of the dye from the disc would constitute an adequate radiological demonstration of a disc rupture. Clinical evaluation, confirmed by the examination of discs injected at autopsy, has failed to substantiate this initial hope. Small tears in the annulus, commonly found in patients over 30 years of age, permit posterior extravasation of the dye, even in the absence of a disc rupture. However, some significance can be placed on the reproduction of clinically experienced symptoms. Reproduction of sciatic pain on injecting a disc is powerful evidence that the level of disc rupture has been found.

Since discography is such an integral part of the chemonucleolysis procedure, it is discussed in more detail in Chapter 10.

CT SCAN

With increasing sophistication of CAT scanners, it is now possible to demonstrate with reasonable accuracy the presence of a ruptured disc (Fig. 6.16). As dosimetry, technique, and software improve, CT scanning will play an increasing role in the diagnosis of an HNP. So in turn will myelography and venography ultimately assume a subordinate role. It is

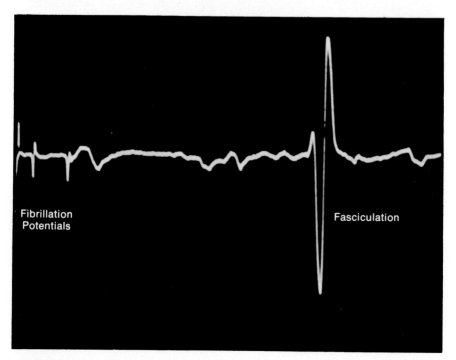

Figure 6.15. A drawing of normal and abnormal electromyographic changes.

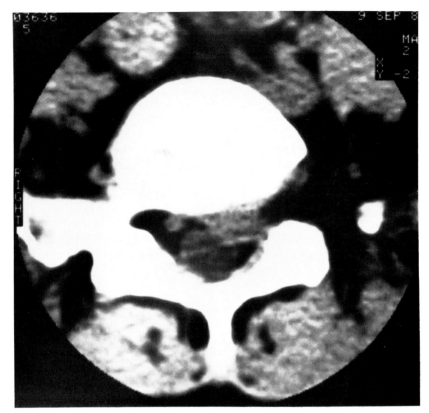

Figure 6.16. CT scan showing an HNP L5-S1, left.

now possible, in some patients, to confirm the clinical impression of root compression with noninvasive CT scan. Combining the CT scan with the technique of lateral discography for the intradiscal injection of chymo-papain, makes the management of an HNP possible without injecting or exposing the spinal canal. This subject will be discussed at greater length in Chapter 10.

NERVE ROOT INFILTRATION

Nerve root infiltration with local anesthetic has proven to be an accurate means of localizing the level of symptomatic root involvement. If, on clinical evaluation, it appears that the patient is suffering from an L5 lesion, the needle is placed in the L5-S1 foramen and 0.5 ml of water-soluble contrast material is injected. If the needle is correctly placed in the root sleeve, the dye will assume a tubular configuration (Fig. 6.17). If the needle is incorrectly placed, the dye will diffuse irregularly and the needle must be repositioned. Originally the technique was used for demonstrating the radiological type of apophysial compression present.

However, the x-ray changes are not of significance in this mode of investigation. The important finding is the abolition of pain on injection of local anesthetic.

The function of the contrast material is just to make sure that the needle has been correctly placed. Once this is verified, 3 ml of 0.5% marcaine is injected and the accuracy of the injection tested by noting the area of sensory loss produced in the lower limb. Abolition of the clinically experienced pain indicates that the root injected is the root involved.

When injecting the first sacral root (Fig. 6.17), the needle is placed in the first sacral dorsal foramen and is pushed forward to emerge through the first ventral foramen. It is at this site that the dye is injected. This is most easily accomplished by using two needles. The first needle is placed down to the top of the ala of the sacrum and is used as a guide. The second 18 gauge needle is inserted at a 45° angle to the first and is advanced toward the first sacral foramen. A pre-bent 26 gauge needle is now passed through the first needle into the foramen and the nerve root

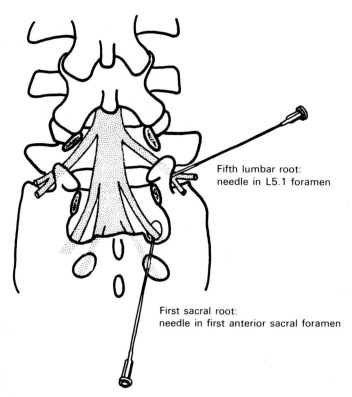

Fifth lumbar root:
needle in L5.1 foramen

First sacral root:
needle in first anterior sacral foramen

Figure 6.17.   Diagram to show the placement of needles for the infiltration of the fifth lumbar and first sacral nerve roots.

can now be injected. Total abolition of pain by the injection of a single nerve root indicates that a simple decompression of the root is all that is required.

Diagnostic nerve root infiltration is most commonly used in the assessment of root involvement in spinal stenosis or in revision surgery where other localizing tests are not reliable.

SUMMARY

When presented with a patient suffering from sciatic-like leg pain, it is encumbent upon the clinician to consider the following points:

1. Is this sciatic-like pain referred pain or pain from some other cause such as vascular claudication?
2. Is this sciatic pain radicular pain and, if so, what evidence is there of root tension, root irritation, and impairment of root conduction?
3. If the pain is radicular pain, is it due to an extradural mass, such as a ruptured disc, or is it due to nerve root compression associated with a spinal stenosis?
4. What root is involved?
5. What disc level is involved?

The diagnosis should be made clinically, and ancillary tests should be used solely as a means of confirmation, not only of the diagnosis, but also of the nerve root involved.

The only patients suitable for treatment by chemonucleolysis are those in whom the sciatic pain is due to compression of an emerging lumbar nerve root by a ruptured disc, in whom the pain usually extends below the knee and is associated with marked root tension. These points will be further emphasized in the section dealing with the indications for chemonucleolysis.

References

1. Kelsey JL: An epidemiological study of acute herniated lumbar intervertebral discs. *Rheumatol Rehabil* 14:144, 1975.
2. Sicard JL: Roentgenologic eploration of the central nervous system with iodized oil (Lipiodol). *Arch Neurol Psychiatry* 16:420, 1926.
3. Mason MS, Raaf J: Complication of Pantopaque myelography: Case report and review. *J Neurosurg* 19:302, 1962.
4. Howland WJ, Curry JL: Experimental studies of Pantopaque arachnoiditis. I. Animal studies. *Radiology* 87:253, 1966.

CHAPTER 7

Pain and Disability

There are no words in the English language that adequately describe pain. The patient can only describe the disability it causes. "The pain in my leg is so severe that I can't make beds and I can't do any vacuum cleaning." The patient is not describing the pain; she is describing her reaction to it. Pain is an experience, often initiated by a physical lesion but always modified by the patient's emotional makeup.

The clinician must be aware of this and must be capable of assessing the significance of the emotional content in the total disability. Of the many causes of failure to respond to chemunocleolysis, the surgeon's failure to recognize a nonorganic or psychogenic disability is high on the list.

The purpose of this chapter is to present a simplified approach to assessment of nonorganic or psychogenic pain. The concepts presented in this chapter are very simple, but very worthwhile to the clinician assessing patients with a complaint of spinal pain on a daily basis. With these concepts and the basic tools of our trade (the history and physical examination), it should be possible for the clinician to at least suspect a nonorganic or psychogenic component to a back disability. With this recognition it is hoped the clinician will obtain help from others more skilled in the evaluation of nonorganic reactions, instead of embarking on that inevitable downhill course of hospital admission, borderline myelographic findings, and a chemonucleolysis which in such instances has a very high risk of failure.

Most patients presenting with pain in the low back have a local organic basis for their disability and can be managed with standard nonsurgical measures such as rest, medication, deep heat, manipulation, and/or appropriate exercises. However, at some time in a musculoskeletal specialty practice, a patient with nonorganic back pain is seen.

The patient may be recognized when he describes a pain with unusual qualities, when he relates emotional symptoms, and when the physical examination reveals either bizarre physical findings or no organic cause for the disability. If the pain is not initially recognized as nonorganic, the cause of the pain will then proceed to elude standard investigations and defy standard physical treatment measures. The true nature of the pain may continue unrecognized until the judicial process has dealt with the claim for financial compensation for the pain and the patient ceases to appear for treatment. All in all, the patient with unrecognized nonorganic spinal pain can become a frustrating problem.

CLASSIFICATION AND DEFINITIONS

A classification of spinal pain is outlined in Table 7.1. Nonorganic spinal pain is obviously back pain with no organic cause. Many terms

Table 7.1
Classification of Spinal Pain

I. ORGANIC SPINAL PAIN
  A. Referred causes
    i. Abdominal aneurysm
    ii. Genitourinary conditions
    iii. Gastrointestinal conditions
    etc.
  B. Local causes
    i. Nonmechanical
     1. Infections of bone or disc
     2. Neoplasm (primary or secondary)
     3. Arthritis (*e.g.*, ankylosing spondylitis)
     4. Metabolic (osteopenias)
    ii. Mechanical
     1. Mechanical instability
      Intrinsic to disc: degenerative disc disease
      Extrinsic to disc: facet joint disease
       Spondylolisthesis
       Congenital lumbosacral anomalies
     2. Disruption of anatomical configuration of disc: herniated nucleus pulposus (HNP)
     3. Narrowing of spinal canal
      Spinal stenosis
      Lateral recess stenosis
     4. Postinvasive (investigation, operation) scarring
     5. Soft tissue syndromes: fibrositis
     6. Fractures and dislocations
II. NONORGANIC SPINAL PAIN
  A. Psychosomatic spinal pain
    i. Tension syndrome (fibrositis)
  B. Psychogenic spinal pain
    i. Psychogenic pain
    ii. Psychogenic modification of organic pain
  C. Situational spinal pain
    i. Litigation reaction
    ii. Exaggeration reaction

have been applied to the pain, the most common being "functional back pain."

The following definitions are used in the presentation:

Psychosomatic spinal pain is defined as symptomatic physical change in tissues of the spine which has as its cause anxiety. The expression of anxiety is mediated as a prolonged and exaggerated state that eventually leads to structural change (spasm) in the muscles of the neck or low back.

Psychogenic spinal pain is defined as the conversion or somatization of anxiety into pain referred to the neck or back, unaccompanied by physical change in the tissues of these regions. The pain is variously known in the literature as conversion hysteria, psychogenic regional pain, traumatic or accident neurosis, and hypochondriasis.

The emotional upset brings pains to the back just as it may bring tears to the eyes. The reason for the conversion is found in complex psychodynamic mechanisms beyond the scope of this chapter. The reaction represents a sincere unconscious emotional illness that offers the patient the primary gain of solving inner conflicts, fears, and anxieties. Inherent in the conversion reaction is the concept of suggestion and hypnosis, the importance of which will become evident later in this chapter.

Psychogenic modification of spinal pain is a sincere emotional reaction which modifies the appreciation of an organic pain. Usually, the organic pain by itself would not be disabling, but with the psychogenic modification a significant disability ensues. This psychogenic modification occurs either on the basis of the emotional makeup of the patient or the life situational pressures existent at the time of the organic pain. No associated physical change occurs as a result of anxiety and a conversion reaction may or may not co-exist.

One example is the patient burdened with life situational pressures (mortgage payments, car payments) who, because of his physical illness, feels he cannot sustain the effort necessary to meet these demands. A resulting depression may occur and the symptoms of fatigue, loss of appetite, insomnia, impotence, constipation, etc., so dominate the history that the underlying physical condition is missed. Other examples are the patients with the passive dependent personality, drug or alcoholic dependence or psychosis, who in face of a minor physical problem use their illness to step out of the demands of the real world. Some obsessive-compulsive patients cannot adjust to a minor physical problem, and this personality trait leads them to feel they have a significant disability.

Situational spinal pain is a reaction whereby a patient, through a collection of symptoms, maintains a situation (with potential secondary gain) through overconcern or conscious effort.

The litigation or compensation reaction is defined as overconcern by the patient for present and future health, arising out of a litigious or compensable event that initially affected health. The reaction manifests itself in a patient's complaint of continuing neck or back pain coupled with a concern that, upon formal severence from his claim to compensation, deterioration in health may occur. The patient with this reaction is neither physically nor emotionally ill.

This reaction is not to be confused with litigation or compensation neurosis, terms which the authors find too ambiguous. Like "whiplash," the terms litigation and compensation neurosis have no medical or legal value and should be dropped from our vocabulary. If a patient has a true neurosis arising out of a litigious or compensable event (accident), then those terms listed under psychogenic spinal pain should be used for diagnostic purposes (*e.g.*, traumatic neurosis or accident neurosis). If the patient's disability appears to be based more in his awareness of the commercial value of his symptoms, his reaction should not be legitimized by the use of the term neurosis in conjunction with the words, "litigation," or, "compensation" (thus: litigation reaction).

Exaggeration reactions are attempts by the patient to appear ill or magnify an existent illness. "Malingering" is a term frequently applied to the reaction and is defined as "the conscious alteration of health for gain."

As will be described below, it is possible for the physician to detect effort to magnify, but it is not proper for him to assign motives (gain) to the patient. The lawyer may cast aspersions and doubts on the plaintiff's motives (gain), but he is in no position to clinically detect effort to magnify or exaggerate which may be conscious effort by the patient. The choice of the word, "malingering," thus implies proficiency in two professions, an uncommon occurrence. For this reason, the terms, "malingering" and "conscious effort," are best not used by the physician when discussing nonorganic spinal pain.

Alteration of health in order to deceive, to evade responsibility, or to derive gain does occur. Those who would deny its occurrence deny the existence of human nature. The patient who tries to alter or reproduce symptoms or signs of a spinal problem may do so in a number of ways:

1. Pretension: No physical illness exists and the patient willfully fabricates symptoms and signs. Not infrequent in the military during wartime, it is a rare civilian event.
2. Exaggeration: Symptoms and signs of a spinal disability are magnified to represent more than they really are.
3. Perseveration: Symptoms and signs that were once present have ceased to exist, but are continued by the patient.
4. Allegation: Genuine disability is present, but the patient fraudulently ascribes these to some cause, associated with gain, knowing that in fact his condition is of different origin.

Civilian nonorganic situational spinal pain is usually the exaggeration or perseveration type. Pretension and allegation are uncommon forms of gainful alteration of health in civilian practice. Like the patient with the litigation reaction, these patients are not emotionally ill nor physically ill. However, they differ from the litigation reaction in that they are attempting to demonstrate physical illness through the effort of exaggeration or perseveration. The reason for this effort is usually, but not always, found in secondary financial gain.

In presenting this classification, we do not wish to imply that each nonorganic reaction can be placed in a pigeonhole. The areas between these three basic classes of nonorganic disorders are gray and overlap. Most patients will tend to fall more towards one class than another.

CLINICAL DESCRIPTION
Psychosomatic Back Pain

The psychosomatic phenomenon of muscle spasm arising out of tension states usually affects the neck, but may affect the low back. It should be known as the "orthopaedic ulcer," but more often is given the label of fibrositis. The patient with this problem is overtly strained and tense, as evidenced by facial expression. They are fidgety and restless and may sit on the edge of the chair while they wring their hands. Some of these patients will place their hands on their neck or back during the history and literally wring the area while describing the pain. They have a general feeling of restlessness and a specific feeling of a tightness in their neck with associated sensations of cracking and a constant feeling of the need to stretch out the neck and shoulder muscles. The pain is not specifically mechanical but does tend to accumulate with the day's activity, especially when that activity is carried out in the tension-producing environment (e.g., work).

The pain typically responds to chiropratic or physiotherapeutic intervention, but relief is usually temporary, a fact that makes the patient vulnerable to those practitioners of these arts who specialize in prolonged care.

Physical examination reveals a good range of movement in the affected part with a complaint of pain only if movement is done too quickly or carried to extremes. The significant physical finding is the presence of firm, tender muscles when the affected part is examined in a position of rest. The patient may be able to demonstrate the "cracking" to the touch or auditory perception of the examiner.

No evidence of nerve root involvement exists in the associated extremities. Skin tenderness, the significance of which is explained below, is not a usual finding.

Psychogenic Back Pain

The patient with psychogenic spinal pain is emotionally ill. These patients often have a history of past illnesses replete with emotional problems. It follows that the history of present illness contains a preponderance of emotional symptoms and the description of the pain will not be typical of any organic condition. The patient is convinced that he is ill and that conviction extends to the frequent demand for consultations with numerous doctors. Considerable financial hardship and aggravation will occur in some cases when these consultations take the patient great distances from and to major clinics or spas throughout the world. Throughout their constant demand for care these patients notice times when their symptoms do improve. This is due to the institution of some new form of treatment that affects the patient through suggestion or hypnosis, a fact that makes placebo trial of little value in the evaluation of these problems.

It follows that because these patients are emotionally ill, no causative organic problem will be found on physical examination. The conversion reaction is associated with an upset in body image appreciation such that a topographical unit (the neck or back), indifferent to matters of innervation or anatomical relationship, will contain physical findings of skin tenderness and dulled sensory appreciation (1). The somatization infrequently reaches the stage of weakness with wasting and depression of all the reflexes in the contiguous part, e.g., an arm or a leg.

However, the important observation on physical examination of this patient is the paucity of physical findings, which separates him from the magnifier and exaggerator who by definition has many "physical" findings.

Psychogenic Modification of Organic Pain

Of all the nonorganic causes of spinal pain, the patient who psychogenically modifies organic pain presents the most difficult diagnostic and therapeutic challenge. It is usual that the organic disability by itself would not be disabling. Thus, the historical and physical component of the disability related to the organicity is not significant. Those findings indicative of a physical illness will be appropriate and a quantitative guide to the extent of physical illness. However, the life situational pressures or the personality of the patient modifies the disability to a significant point. As well, the psychogenic reaction interferes with response to treatment and leads to persistence of the disability. In a surgical practice, this failure to respond to conservative treatment is the classic indication for operative intervention. If the surgeon fails to recognize that the failure to respond to treatment is due to a psychogenic disability, he will gradually build a practice containing a number of spinal surgery failures. Psychogenic modifications are commonly seen in the patient with an inadequate personality. By definition the patient's personality may limit advancement up the social, educational, and occupational ladder and confine him to the unskilled worker classification. Some of these patients can be found in the Workman's Compensation Board population and may be one of the reasons for poorer results to treatment sometimes obtained in the Board patient.

They are seen with a minor physical problem (*e.g.*, back strain), yet have a total disability. All attempts at treatment fail to return the patient to the work force. Frequent office visits reinforce the disability for the patient. If the doctor fails to recognize this maladaptive reaction and reinforcement, he may add a scar to, or stick a needle into the back, which will not help the patient in any way.

Other psychogenic modifications come about through drug addiction and alcoholic dependence. Occasionally psychotic behavior will convert a minor physical problem into a prolonged disability.

Physical examination will reveal the nature and extent of the physical impairment. It is usual, but not universal, that the physical impairment by itself would not be significantly disabling. The loss of movement in the back is minor, the limitation of straight leg raising is minimal, and the neurological changes are of questionable significance. In the face of repeated assessments and a continuing statement of disability, the patient's minor physical problem may become magnified in the mind of the clinician who does not assess personality and life situational factors.

Situational Spinal Pain

LITIGATION REACTION

This patient is neither physically nor emotionally ill. Thus, few emotional symptoms will be present on historical examination. The patient is in the process of litigation or under the care of the Workman's Compensation Board. These patients often state that they do not care about the litigious or compensation issue yet they also state that they are afraid to settle or return to work for fear that further illness will develop. Their continuing complaints are rather vague and should not be incapacitating. If they are on treatment, they are not improving.

Physically there may be an increased awareness of the part as manifested by skin tenderness in the affected area, but there is no organic illness detectable and no attempt to exaggerate or magnify a disability.

MAGNIFICATION EXAGGERATION REACTION

Some or most of the following historical characteristics will be obtained from this patient. The most obvious historical point is the secondary gain situation which usually involves the fault of someone else and/or payment of financial compensation. Other secondary gain situations can occur. The initiating event is usually a trivial or minor incident. There may be a latent period of hours or days between the incident and the onset of symptoms during which time the patient speaks to friends and relatives and learns the commercial value of the injury.

The patient describes the pain with some degree of indifference as evidenced by a smile or a laugh when describing his severe disability. He is vague in describing and localizing the pain, giving the examiner the impression of someone struggling to remember a dream. Specificity and elaboration require memory for repetition, a quality not present to a significant degree in this type of patient. The individual wishes you to believe this pain is unique and severe. This attempt to have you believe in the pain is often accompanied by a salesman-like attitude with many examples of the disability spontaneously listed. Inability to achieve sexual satisfaction is usually at the top of the list.

In spite of the trivial initiating event, the disability may have been present for a long time. Three types of treatment patterns occur:
A. The patient follows a "straight line" course of treatment; he does not respond to the standard treatment nor to the suggestion and hypnosis of treatment, i.e., he does not improve or he gets worse.
B. The patient is not on treatment because he is allergic to all medications prescribed, he suffocates in the neck or back braces, or he becomes ill in a physiotherapy setting.
C. The patient is not on treatment because he has not sought treatment.

Certain behavioral patterns become evident after seeing a number of these patients. Some never appear for appointments in spite of weeks of notification. Others appear late for the appointment and do not apologize or state indifferently that the traffic was heavy. There may be an attempt to manipulate your feelings with a compliment about your reputation or your office. There may be an effort to play one doctor against another by making false statements about the doctor. Finally, hostility may appear during the assessment. A patient sincerely ill will not be aware or afraid of exposure and will not be hostile unless provoked. A patient exaggerating a disability is suspicious. He may start out hostile, but the usual pattern is one of developing hostility as discrepancies in the history and physical examination are exposed. Examiners are advised, for obvious reasons, not to precipitate this final behavioral pattern.

The patient who is magnifying or exaggerating a disability can only be exposed through an adequate physical examination. Those physicians who do not physically examine patients will not recognize this reaction, which may explain the reluctance of the psychiatric community to accept this clinical entity.

The physical findings of magnification or exaggerated reaction are classified into those demonstrating acting behavior, those indicative of anticipatory behavior, and those that fail to support the patient's claim to illness.

Acting Behavior

Effort to exaggerate a disability requires acting by the patient. This acting may be general in nature such as the Academy Award performances put on by some patients as they moan and groan through the examination, walk around the examining room with their eyes closed, and either reach for objects to support themselves or reach for their painful area. The incongruity of this acting behavior may be evident when the patient mounts the examining table with considerable ease and/or dresses within minutes of the examination and smiles and waves goodby as he leaves the office.

Specific examples of acting behavior are the rigid back, the reduction in straight leg raising (SLR), tender skin, and the paralyzed insensitive extremity. The acting nature of these physical efforts can be demonstrated through the use of distraction testing (Table 7.2). Using nonpainful, nonemotional, and nonsurprising examination techniques, it is possible not only to change the acting behavior but also to *demonstrate normal physical function*. It is the authors' opinion that proper distraction testing that abolishes an acted physical finding and demonstrates normal physical function is a method of demonstrating magnification exaggeration behavior.

The best distraction test is simple observation of the patient as he gets undressed and moves about the examining room. Other more specific methods of distraction testing are outlined in Figure 7.1.

Table 7.2
Distraction Testing

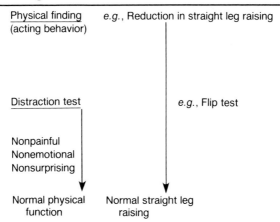

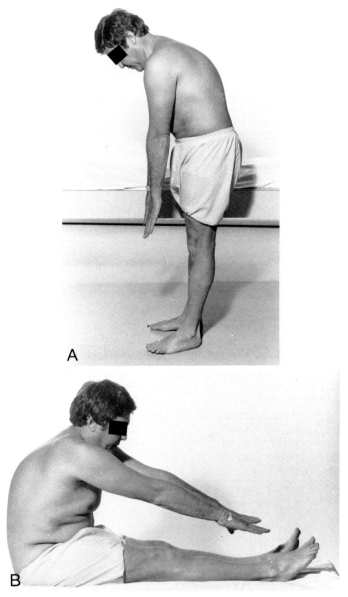

Figure 7.1. *A* and *B,* distraction test. Patient demonstrates no lumbar flexion while standing, yet good lumbar flexion while sitting. Although not evident in this picture, one can also observe reversal of the lumbar lordosis in the sitting position.

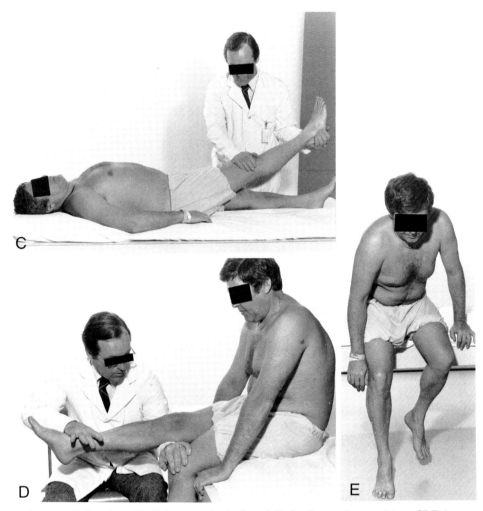

Figure 7.1. *C* to *E*, distraction test. *C* and *D*, In the supine position, SLR is reduced, yet in the sitting position, SLR is 90°. *E*, a patient who has demonstrated a diffuse weakness of the right lower extremity would not ordinarily leave the examining table by leading with that extremity.

Varying degrees of acting behavior occur in different patients. In general, the more sophisticated the patient, the more sophisticated is the acting behavior and the more sophisticated the examiner must be.

Anticipatory Behavior

The second group of physical findings in this reaction represent antic-ipation on the part of the patient to the test situations. This anticipatory behavior leads to an appropriate response by the patient in an attempt to indicate illness. These tests are illustrated in Figure 7.2.

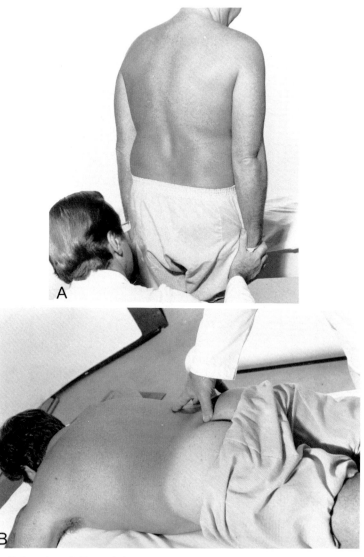

Figure 7.2. *A* and *B*, anticipatory test. *A*, simulated back movement. In this test, the patient is rotated through the hips and knees, but the back is neither flexed nor extended. A patient with a magnification-exaggeration reaction may complain of *back* pain, even though the spine has undergone no postural change. Reproduction of *leg* pain during this test may indicate sciatic irritation aggravated by the pyriformis tendon. *B*, a patient with a magnification-exaggeration reaction, anticipating pain anywhere in the low back, will complain of pain when pressure is applied over the body of the sacrum. Patients with organic low back pain will *not* have tenderness over the body of the sacrum except in the case of a sacral tumor.

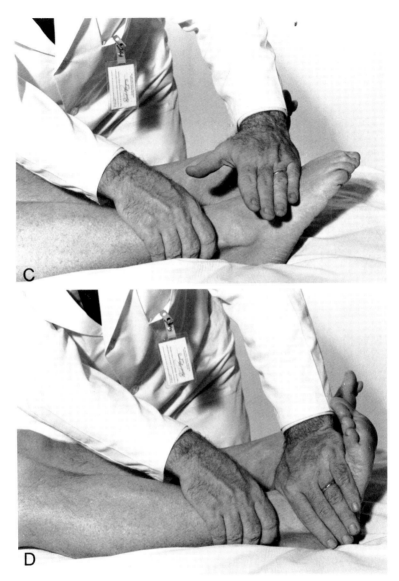

Figure 7.2. *C* and *D*, anticipatory test. *C*, a patient wishing to demonstrate weakness of dorsiflexion often signifies it with toe flexion. *D*, normal position of the toes during testing for dorsiflexion weakness.

Contradictory Clinical Evidence

Statements by the patient to the effect that he is unable to work may not be supported by clinical observations. Some patients will state they are unable to drive, yet will have driven by themselves great distances to get to the examination. Some patients will state that they require frequent medication, yet will arrive from great distances without their medication. The patient who claims to be continuously wearing a collar or brace should show signs of this wear on his body and the appliance. Patients with callouses on their hands and knees contradict their story of a prolonged inability to work. Other evidence of work may be in the form of paint stains or a particular distribution to their sunburn. Patients with nicotine stains on a grossly paralyzed limb should start to demonstrate similar stains on the opposite hand. Finally, those patients who demonstrate a prolonged and profound weakness in an extremity will not have associated wasting of that extremity.

Further assistance in assessing these reactions may be sought with the use of the Pentothal pain study, psychometric testing, and the pain drawing.

THE PENTOTHAL PAIN STUDY

The introduction of the thiopental sodium pain assessment by Walters (2) has been of inestimable value in assessing the significance of emotional states and the production of the disability presented by the patient. The basis of this test lies in the fact that, at the stage of light anesthesia, although the patient is unconscious, he is still capable of demonstrating primitive reactions to pain. The patient is anesthetized with thiopental and then allowed to rouse until the corneal reflex returns. At this state of anesthesia, he will withdraw from pinprick and will grimace when a painful stimulus is applied, such as squeezing the tendo achillis. With the patient maintained at this level of anesthesia, maneuvers that were previously painful on clinical examination are reevaluated. If, for example, with the knee held extended, the patient grimaces when the leg has been raised just 20°, this finding may be taken as irrefutable evidence of significant root tension regardless of the presence of any associated emotional breakdown. If, on the other hand, at the stage of anesthesia where the patient will withdraw from pinprick, straight leg raising which was only 20° on clinical examination can now be carried out to 90° without any response from the patient, the clinician may safely conclude that there is no evidence of root tension and that the patient's disability is due to his emotional reaction rather than to any organic source of pain.

If the patient previously had the diffuse stocking-type of hypoesthesia, at this stage of narcosis he will withdraw his limb when it is pricked by a pin. If, however, in addition to the hysterical response there is a physiogenically induced root compression, then the patient will not show any response on pricking the skin over the dermatome of the root involved.

PSYCHOMETRIC TESTING

Psychometric testing is a simple though rough guide to a patient's emotional health and is useful to those physicians and surgeons who are

Table 7.3
Symptoms and Signs Suggesting a Nonorganic Component to Patient's
Disability

SYMPTOMS
1. Pain is multifocal in distribution and nonmechanical (present at rest)
2. Entire extremity is painful, numb, and/or weak
3. Extremity gives way
4. Treatment response:
   A. No response
   B. "Allergic" to treatment
   C. None on treatment
5. Multiple crisis, multiple hospital admissions/investigations, multiple doctors

SIGNS
1. Tenderness is superficial (skin) or nonanatomical (*e.g.*, over body of sacrum)
2. Simulated movement tests positive
3. Distraction tests positive
4. Whole leg weak or numb
5. Academy Award performance

not familiar with clinical assessment of emotional breakdown, particularly the difficult group of depression. Wiltse and Rocchio (3) demonstrated convincingly that patients with a good emotional profile as shown by Minnesota Multiphasic Personality Inventory (MMPI) studies could be confidently expected to obtain better results following chemonucleolysis than those patients in whom a psychological profile is not obtained.

The pain drawings, popularized by Mooney and Cairns (4) are a simple form of psychometric testing which can be done by the patients themselves while in the waiting room. Patients on the whole do not like answering an MMPI questionnaire. They tend, because of the nature of the questions asked, to regard this as an affront to their intelligence and emotional integrity. They resent this and regard it as an invasion of their privacy.

However, they do not mind doing a pain drawing as they regard this as cooperating with the physician in keeping an adequate record of their symptoms.

CONCLUSION

Every human attends the school of survival. Sometimes the lessons lead patients to modify or magnify a physical disability at a conscious or unconscious level. *These reactions will not dissolve away with chemonucleolysis.* But one word of caution—the presence of one of these nonorganic reactions does not immunize the patient from an organic condition such as a herniated nucleus pulposus. The art of medicine is truly tested when the surgeon faces the difficult clinical situation of a patient with an organic low back pain who modifies the disability with a nonorganic reaction of tension, hysteria, depression, etc. More often the surgeon opts for the "chance" that the magic of chemonucleolysis will resolve the problem when in fact he should be asking for help from his nonsurgical colleagues to separate the organic from the nonorganic.

Table 7.3 summarizes the symptoms and signs suggesting a nonorganic component to the patient's disability. If a few of these clinical features are present, stop, do not invade, call for help.

References

1. Waddell G, McCulloch JA, Kummel E, *et al.*: Non-organic physical signs in low-back pain. *Spine* 5:117, 1980.
2. Walters A: Psychogenic regional pain alias hysterical pain. *Brain* 84:1, 1961.
3. Wiltse LL, Rocchio PO: Preoperative psychological tests as predictors of success of chemonucleolysis in the treatment of the low back syndrome. *J Bone Joint Surg* 57A:478, 1975.
4. Mooney V, Cairns D: Management in the patient with chronic low back pain. *Orthop Clin North Am* 9:543, 1978.

CHAPTER 8

Chymopapain—Chemistry and Tissue Reaction

Chymopapain is one of the proteolytic enzymes contained in crude "papain," a mixture derived from papaya latex, in turn derived from the papaya plant. After considerable investigation, it has been found to have a narrower tissue specificity, lower activity, faster electrophoretic mobility, and higher solubility at neutral pH than crude papain (1). For these reasons it has been selected as probably the best proteolytic enzyme for dissolution of nuclear disc material.

The concept of using proteolytic enzymes to digest dead tissue has been around for decades. Natives of tropical countries knew for years that if they scratched the skin of a papaya plant, they could obtain a papain-rich latex to treat eczema, warts, ulcers, and other types of foul sores.

Thomas (2) was the first to describe the selective effect of papain on hyaline cartilage when he injected it intravenously into immature rabbits and noticed their ears wilt and droop. Hirsch (3) was the first to suggest, in 1959, that a proteolytic enzyme might be injected into protruded nuclear pulposus to relieve the clinical symptoms. Smith (4), after considerable laboratory and clinical experimentation centered around numerous enzymes, was the first to report its experimental use in *Nature* in 1963 and its clinical use in 1964 (5).

ACTION
In Vitro

Think of the nucleus pulposus as a lattice of collagen fibrils interlaced in a mucopolysaccharide-protein (proteoglycan) gel. When slices of nucleus are incubated in chymopapain, there is a visible collapse of the structure as the proteoglycan is hydrolyzed. This leaves a network of collagen fibers in milky solution (6). The collagenous elements are recovered largely undissolved after 12 hours of incubation. After analyzing the insoluble residues after digestion, Stern (1) has demonstrated that chymopapain attacks mainly the noncollagenous proteoglycan portion of the nucleus pulposus. The initiating binding mechanism that allows this specific attack probably relates to the fact that at physiological pH, chymopapain bears a strong positive charge and proteoglycan is negatively charged.

Stern also demonstrated a smaller degree of chymopapain binding in displaced lumbar disc material which reflected its lower content of proteoglycan. This early observation explains one of the mechanisms of failure to dissolve a sequestered disc; *i.e.*, even if chymopapain can reach

97

a sequestered disc, it may have no effect on the disc fragment because of its predominantly collagenous nature.

Finally, Stern's work clearly demonstrated that the dissolution of the nucleus was proportional to the concentrate (volume) of enzyme. Use of too little enzyme precludes a maximal effect on nuclear material.

With the disruption of the proteoglycan complex of the nucleus, the water-binding capacity is impaired, in turn reducing the volume and intradiscal pressure of the nucleus pulposus.

In Vivo

Garvin and co-workers (7) conducted extensive pharmacological and toxicological studies in experimental animals. They showed that low doses of chymopapain effectively and selectively removed the nucleus pulposus of dogs and rabbits. They noted narrowing of the injected intervertebral disc space, both grossly and on x-ray. With effective doses of chymopapain, most or all of the components of the nucleus pulposus disappeared. The peripheral, more fibrous portion of the annulus and surrounding structures such as dura, nerve roots, bone, and ligaments were unaffected.

Grossly observable effects on the nucleus pulposus did not become evident until about 24 hours after injection, regardless of the dosage used, and were not maximal until at least 4 to 8 days. Of interest was their inability to harvest any unspent chymopapain immediately after injection. They concluded that chymopapain was immediately bound to proteoglycan and instantly hydrolyzed the proteoglycan. The delayed appearance of gross changes *in vivo* probably resulted from a slow absorption of the reaction products from the disc related to the relative avascular nature of the disc.

TOXICITY

Garvin and co-workes (7) demonstrated that intradiscal and epidural doses of chymopapain up to 100 times in excess of the effective dose were well tolerated in rabbits and dogs. Maximally tolerated doses of chymopapain injected intravenously, intradiscally, and epidurally did not produce any acute gross or microscopic pathological disturbance in the intrathecal space, such as subarachnoid hemorrhage or arachnoiditis, and did not cause delayed neurotoxicity during periods of observation up to 3 months. Lethal doses also produced minimal local reaction with death resulting from systemic hemorrhage.

On the other hand, marked subarachnoid hemorrhage and high mortality was seen following the *intrathecal* administration of chymopapain.

Garvin's work appeared to establish the safety of chymopapain injection. However, Shealy (8) presented contrary evidence after applying 10 mg of chymopapain to the exposed dura of cats. He claimed to have produced massive subarachnoid hemorrhage and death in some cats and subarachnoid thickening in some survivors. Ford (9), Gesler (10), Wiltse *et al.* (11), and we (12) repeated Shealy's experimental work and could not reproduce his results. We conclude again that chymopapain applied to the exposed dura of dogs and cats produced neither subarachnoid hemorrhage nor epidural scarring.

Rydevik and co-workers (13), using chymopapain on rabbit tibial nerve as an experimental model, noted impairment of barrier function of the perineural sheath and increased permeability of the intraneural micro-vessels resulting in intraneural edema formation. Long-term conse-quences were degeneration of nerve fibers and formation of intraneural fibrosis, requiring an increased threshold voltage for eliciting action potentials. Their concern was with leakage of chymopapain at the time of injection producing a "chemical rhizotomy" effect on the nerve tissue in the annulus and nerve roots. In reply Wiltse (14) has pointed out that spinal nerve roots are covered by dura and circulation is intradural, in contrast to the rabbit tibial nerve Rydevik used. In addition, chymopa-pain is strongly bound to substrates in the disc, so that concentrations of chymopapain leaking out of the intradiscal space would be much less than the dose used by Rydevik. Further, not all injections of chymopapain leak out of the intradiscal space. Finally, Wiltse and co-workers (11) restated their experimental work on chymopapain, bathing nerves in the epidural space following which there were no changes in the intrathecal elements, the dura, or the epidural elements on the spinal nerves. Wiltse concluded that the experimental model used by Rydevik was probably not relevant to intradiscal injection of chymopapain. Support for this position is evident in the over 7000 injections done in this center with no chemical nerve toxicity demonstrated.

There is universal agreement among all investigators that chymopa-pain in the intrathecal space has potentially devastating effects. Chy-mopapin dissolves the basement membanes in the small vessels of the pia-arachnoid to produce a subarachnoid hemorrhage which in laboratory animals was often fatal. We noticed that immediate decompression of the subarachnoid space (opening the dura) when chymopapain was injected intrathecally reduced fatalities significantly. Because of the intrathecal toxicity of chymopapain it is not possible to use the standard midline discographic approach. To avoid penetrating the dura, the lateral approach (Chapter 10) must be used for chemonucleolysis. Often, at the time of discography or discometry, test material will leak through a rent in the annulus, but the collagenous dural sheath obviously serves as an effective barrier to chymopapain leaking into the intrathecal space. Related is the requirement of 24 hours delay between myelography and chemonucleolysis, especially if myelography has been difficult and en-tailed the use of a large bore needle to instill oil-based contrast material. This delay will allow any dural rent to seal and preclude inadvertent leakage of chymopapain into the subarachnoid space.

Chymopapain, as package by Baxter (Discase) contains other compo-nents to protect the enzyme. Sulfhydryl (—SH) groups are required for activity and the enzyme is, therefore, inactivated by heavy metals and oxygen. Disodium edetate is added to combine with heavy metals and cysteine to maintain sulfur amino acids in —SH form.

In solution, in the absence of other protein substrates, the enzyme eventually digests itself, causing progressive loss of activity. As with all enzymes, the rate of hydrolysis increases rapidly as the temperature is raised. Therefore, chymopapain solutions should not be kept at room temperature for more than 30 minutes before injection and should not be stored after mixing for longer than 5 hours, even if refrigerated.

SUMMARY OF SEQUENCE OF EVENTS AFTER INJECTION OF CHYMOPAPAIN INTO NUCLEUS PULPOSUS

Immediately on injection into the disc, the enzyme:

a. Depolymerizes (hydrolyzes) soluble high molecular weight mucopolysaccharide-protein complexes (proteoglycans), the action occurring in the first few seconds to hours.
b. Binds to less soluble components instantly—thus, there is little left to affect the annulus or spill out into surrounding tissue or circulation.
c. The dissolved components of nucleus in combination with the inactivated chymopapain diffuse rapidly out of the disc into the circulation.

It is a combination of chymopapain and soluble disc components that form the milky fluid which often refluxes from the disc space immediately after injection.
d. Residues of the original enzyme may remain in the disc to catalyze slow decomposition of less soluble noncollagenous residues over a period of several hours.
e. Further diffusion of residual degraded nucleus pulposus and chymopapain out of the disc space occurs over a period of several days.

FATE OF INJECTED CHYMOPAPAIN

Most chymopapain is immediately spent on hydrolysis of the nucleus.

Some of the enzyme or its immunologically reactive fragments (CIP) is detectable in low concentrations in plasma by radioimmunoassay (17). Because of the inhibitory action of plasma α_2-macroglobulins and low concentrations, it is unlikely that any proteolytic activity of chymopapain is expressed outside the disc.

Finally, antibodies develop within the disc space and residual chymopapain protein is removed completely by proteolysis in the reticuloendothelial system. Simply stated, chymopapain's activity is immediate, with no lasting proteolytic activity possible.

RECONSTITUTION OF DISC

Brown (15) in Florida and Wiltse (16) in California have reported reconstitution of disc height years after chymopapain injection (Fig. 8.1).

This may be explained by Garvin's work, using young (9 months old) non-chrondrodystrophoid beagle pups, and injecting a minimal dose of chymopapain. At various intervals after injection, he noticed decreased

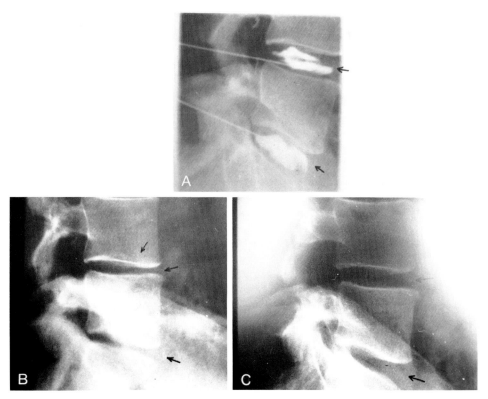

Figure 8.1.   L4-L5 and L5-S1 disc spaces (*A*) before chemonucleolysis (at time of discography, (*B*), 2 months after chemonucleolysis, and (*C*) 3 years after chemonucleolysis. After narrowing of both disc spaces at 2 months, the disc spaces have reconstituted to normal height at 3 years. (Courtesy of Leon Wiltse.)

disc width due to a decrease in nuclear cells and noncellular substances. But with these low doses of chymopapain, scattered cells were noticed still persisting in the nucleus. Twenty-four months later a number of these immature dogs showed reestablishment of disc height which must have been due to regeneration of nucleus pulposus through remaining viable chrondrocytes. The use of larger doses of chymopapain (2 ml, 4000 units, 8 mg) has reduced reconstitution in our series to a negligible level.

In summary, chymopapain can effectively dissolve nuclear material of the intervertebral disc by breaking down noncollagenous ground substance. Providing no intrathecal injection occurs, there is a wide margin of safety between the effective therapeutic dose and toxic side effects (estimated 100:1). The doses used for chemonucleolysis thus have no effect on surrounding ligaments, bone, nervous tissue, dura, or large blood vessels. Injection of adequate amounts of chymopapain will probably prevent reconstitution of the disc through reformation of nuclear material.

References

1. Stern IJ: Biochemistry of chymopapain. *Clin Orthop* 67:42, 1969.
2. Thomas L: Reversible collapse of rabbit ears after intravenous papain and prevention by cortisone. *J Csp Med* 104:245, 1956.
3. Hirsch C: Studies on the pathology of low back pain. *Bone Joint Surg* 41:237, 1959.
4. Smith L, *et al.*: Enzyme dissolution of nucleus pulposus. *Nature* 198:1398, 1963.
5. Smith L: Enzyme dissolution of the nucleus pulposus in humans. *JAMA* 187:137, 1964.
6. Stern IJ, Smith L: Dissolution by chymopapain in vitro of tissue from normal or prolapsed intervertebral discs. *Clin Orthop* 50:269, 1967.
7. Garvin PJ, Jennings RB, Smith L, *et al*: Chymopapain: A pharmacologic and toxicologic evaluation in experimental animals. *Clin Orthop* 41:204, 1965.
8. Shealy CN: Tissue reactions to chymopapain in cats. *J Neurosurg* 26:327, 1967.
9. Ford LT: Experimental study of chymopapain in cats. *Clin Orthop* 67:68, 1969.
10. Gesler RM: Pharmacologic properties of chymopapain. *Clin Orthop* 67:47, 1969.
11. Wiltse LL, Widell EH, Hansen AY: Chymopapain chemonucleolysis in lumbar disc disease. *JAMA* 231:474, 1975.
12. Macnab I, *et al.*: Chemonucleolysis. *Can J Surg* 14:280, 1971.
13. Rydevik B, *et al.*: Effects of chymopapain on nerve tissue. *Spine* 1:137, 1976.
14. Wiltse LL: Letter to the Editor: *Spine* 2:237, 1977.
15. Brown M: Personal communication.
16. Wiltse LL: Personal communication.
17. Kapsalis J, *et al.*: *J Lab Clin Med* 83:532, 1978.

CHAPTER 9

Selection of Patients for Chemonucleolysis

The authors make no apology for repeating the fact that chemonucle-olysis is only of value in the treatment of those patients in whom the symptom of sciatic pain is due to compromise of a lumbar nerve root by rupture of an intervertebral disc.

Chymopapain will only dissolve nucleus pulposus. It has no direct effect on annulus fibrosis nor does it dissolve osteophytes or scar tissue or relieve emotional strains. Selecting the proper patient for chemonu-cleolysis obviously depends on your clinical ability to recognize the patient with sciatica due to a disc herniation.

THE CLASSIC PRESENTATION

The classic patient presentation will involve a young (25 to 40 years old) man (men:women = 2:1) who may or may not describe a history of injury. Somewhere in the history, presently or in the past, there will be low back pain, but the dominating complaint on presentation will be sciatica, pain in the leg and buttock which is described as a deep boring pain in the buttock, a sharp pain in the thigh, and a cramping vise-like sensation in the calf. Whether the pain is lateral or posterior in the thigh or calf is of little localizing value. The pain may be aggravated by coughing, sneezing, or straining at stool. It may take some time for rest to have any effect on the severity of the pain and that rest is usually sought on the back with the legs propped up on a pillow or stool or by lying on the unaffected side with the hips and knees at 90°. Of localizing value is the paresthetic discomfort that may be present in the foot. The patients will describe it variously as tingling, pins and needles, or burning, and it will follow the lateral border of the foot and heel for first root involvement and the lateral calf and dorsum of the foot for fifth root involvement. Pain in the foot is unusual. The symptom of weakness is also not prevalent unless the neurological root lesion is profound.

On physical examination of the back, there may or may not be scoliosis with the tilt, if present, being away from the side of the lesion. Its absence and tilting toward the side of the lesion are so common (especially the former) that it is a physical finding of limited value. On forward flexion muscle spasm may become evident and the lumbar spine moves very little, maintaining its flattened position. Forward flexion is usually quite limited and accompanied by flexion of the hip and knee on the affected side and forward rotation of the pelvis (effectively rotating the hip externally) (Fig. 6.1).

Straight leg raising (SLR), performed with the patient supine and the hip internally rotated and adducted (slightly) and the knee forced into extension, will usually produce buttock and thigh pain at less than 50% of normal. On occasion straight leg raising will produce additional back pain, calf discomfort, or paresthesia in the foot. Raising the "well leg" may produce pain in the affected leg (usually in the hip) (crossover pain). An early and subtle sign of a disc bulge is the sitting crossover straight leg raising test. With the patient in the sitting position (which increases pressure within the disc space), raising the well leg may cause pain to radiate into the buttock on the symptomatic side.

Pressure over the tibial nerve in the popliteal fossa (bowstring test) may produce radiating thigh and buttock discomfort and occasionally may produce distal radiation of pain and/or paresthesia. In the very acute disc, this test should be done with care as considerable pain may occur at the moment of compression.

Many patients, especially the young, may not show any neurologic signs. When patients are seen with root conduction deficits, as evidenced by impairment of motor power, sensory appreciation, or reflex activity, it is of great value in defining the root involved. With the use of myelography, venography, or CT scanning, the clinical diagnosis and the exact location of the disc herniation can be demonstrated.

Unfortunately, the patients who might benefit from chemonucleolysis do not always present in a classic fashion. Nevertheless, there is a common thread through all of the clinical presentations of sciatica due to a soft disc herniation, and it centers around the dominance of leg pain in the history and its location in the leg, the association of neurological symptoms and signs and limitation of straight leg raising, with or without crossover pain and/or a positive bowstring sign. Without this common clinical thread, it is not good enough to demonstrate a myelographic, venographic, or scan defect, and simply "shoot" the drug.

Thus, we work with the "Rule of 5," a set of criteria that describe the classic patient:

1. Leg pain (including buttock) is the dominant complaint when compared to back pain; it affects one leg only and follows a typical sciatic (or femoral) nerve distribution.
2. Paresthesias in the leg or foot follow a typical dermatomal pattern. (Weakness, if present as a symptom, should follow a myotomal distribution).
3. SLR changes—any one, two, or three of the following:
   a. SLR is less than 50% of normal (when compared to normal or the unaffected opposite leg) and the discomfort so produced is relieved by flexing the knee and is aggravated by dorsiflexing the foot.
   b. Pain crosses over into the affected leg when the well leg is raised.
   c. Bowstring testing causes radiating pain in the leg (see text).
4. Two of four neurological signs are present—reflex alteration, wasting, weakness, or sensory loss. One neurological change by itself does not constitute a positive neurological examination. Some might argue that a depressed ankle reflex alone may be indicative of S1 root involvement, and we would agree except to point out that it is rare to have

this reflex finding isolated from other neurological changes, such as wasting of the calf or slight weakness of plantar flexion or a sensory loss. Certainly the isolated finding of muscle atrophy, and the isolated finding of a sensory loss are not absolute clinical findings of nerve root involvement.

5. Positive ancillary investigations in the form of a water-soluble myelogram, CT scan, or epidural venogram.

Notice that these five criteria are composed of two symptoms, two signs, and one investigation. A patient with all five of these criteria is the classic case of a herniated nucleus pulposus (HNP) causing sciatica and the classic indication for chemonucleolysis. A patient with four of five criteria is also likely to have an HNP and is also likely to respond to chemonucleolysis. The two exceptions in this group are:

a. The younger patient who often will show no neurological signs.
b. The older patient whose SLR test tends to be less reduced than the younger patient.

We have stated in past publications (1, 2) that patients with three of five of these criteria may have a disc herniation but with the advent of CT scanning and water-soluble myelography this statement must be modified. There will be the rare occasion in a young patient when the clinical presentation will exclude any neurological symptoms or signs, *i.e.*, the patient is seen with dominant leg pain, a significant reduction in SLR, and a positive radiculogram or CT scan. That patient probably has an HNP (usually at L5–S1) and will respond to chemonucleolysis. On the other hand, the older patient who is seen with dominant back pain, fifth lumbar root paresthesia, a mild reduction in SLR, minor fifth root neurological changes, and a positive myelogram probably does not have an HNP, but rather a spinal canal or recess stenosis and thus has a high likelihood of failure following chemonucleolysis.

Patients with two or fewer of these criteria are not likely to have an HNP and are not likely to respond to chemonucleolysis.

The criteria again:

2 symptoms: 1. Leg pain > back pain
               2. Specific neurological symptoms (paresthesia)
2 signs: 3. SLR—50% of normal
                  —and/or crossover
                  —and/or positive bowstring test
               4. Two of four neurological signs
1 investigation: 5. Positive-water soluble myelogram
                  —and/or CT scan
                  —and/or venogram.

Notice that discography and electromyography are not part of the investigative criterion. We feel there are too many false positives and negatives in these two investigative steps to be included in the criteria. We are sure this will provoke a lot of disagreement, but these criteria have served us so well that we suggest they be used in selecting patients for chemonucleolysis.

THE ROLE OF THE CT SCAN

At the time of writing this monograph, the gold standard of investigation for an HNP is the water-soluble myelogram (radiculogram). The demonstration of nerve roots with water-soluble contrast material, especially at L5–S1, is so important to the assessment of a patient with sciatica that oil-soluble myelography is of little use. In making this statement we are aware of the limitations of water-soluble contrast material for assessment of pathology at higher spinal levels. If a patient has a negative water-soluble myelogram (Fig. 9.1) because of a short dural sac or a wide space between the dural sac and the L5–S1 disc space, then an epidural myelogram or a CT scan is indicated.

With the increasing sophistication of CT scanners, technique of CT scanning, and radiologists' interpretations, we are in the midst of a shift toward CT scanning as the primary diagnostic step in HNP. We are in agreement with this thrust, but make the following observations as clinicians.

1. Older generation CT scanners are of limited value.
2. You need more than a late generation CT scanner. You also need good technique, especially in getting the gantry angle set properly at L5–S1, and a good radiological interpretation.
3. Your radiologist will not hone his skills without input from you, as a clinician, before CT scanning and after your treatment intervention.
4. CT scanning is of limited value in the patient who has had previous surgery.
5. CT scanning at L4–5 and L5–S1 will not give information about L3–4 and higher thoracolumbar levels where a cauda equina lesion (tumor) may lie (Fig. 9.2).
6. CT scanning will give some indication as to the nature of a disc herniation, but in our experience has not demonstrated the so-called sequestered disc that will not respond to chemonucleolysis (Fig. 9.3, A and B).

The CT scanner is truly a remarkable tool, but enthusiasm for this noninvasive step will swing the pendulum too far into its use as a diagnostic screening test rather than using it in a similar role to myelography, that is to say, used after a decision to operate has been made on clinical assessment. Its function is solely to verify the clinical impression.

LESS THAN CLASSIC PRESENTATIONS
The Lateral Disc Herniation (3, 4)

Most lumbar disc herniations occur in the posterolateral portion of the disc and at L5–S1 will compress the first sacral root. However, a small percentage of disc herniations will occur in the far lateral position and at L5–S1 will compress the fifth lumbar nerve root as it courses through the root canal and foramen. This so-called "wrong level" disc lies outside the boundaries of the spinal canal and in the past eluded investigation and failed detection on limited exploration. Epidural venography will detect these lesions but the real revolution in diagnosis is the CT scan

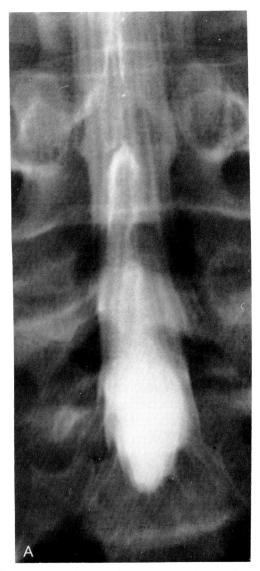

Figure 9.1. *A*, normal anteroposterior myelogram.

(Fig. 9.4). With the advent of this investigative tool these lesions are now readily recognized and the clinical presentation is starting to fall into place.

The patient group tends to be younger than the average age for the classic disc herniation. The leg pain continues to dominate the history and paresthesias are present in approximately 50%. Straight leg raising is characteristically less restricted and in some cases may approach 90°.

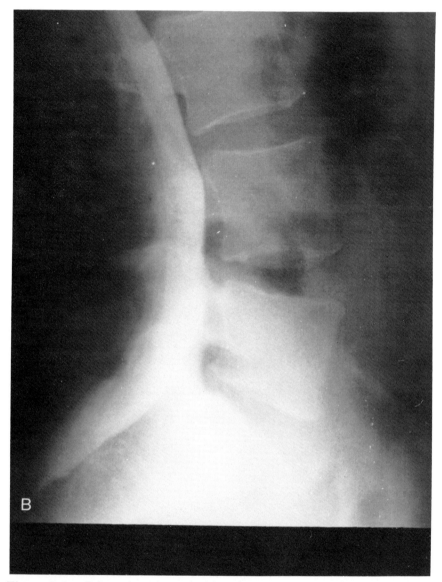

Figure 9.1.   *B,* lateral myelogram with wide insensitive space between the back of the fifth lumbar vertebral body and the anterior aspect of the contrast column.

The neurological lesion is often pronounced which fits with the explusion of material into the foramen where limited room allows for maximal root compression. Compression of the nerve root at this level (spinal ganglion or distal) does not seem to produce any unusual symptoms such as

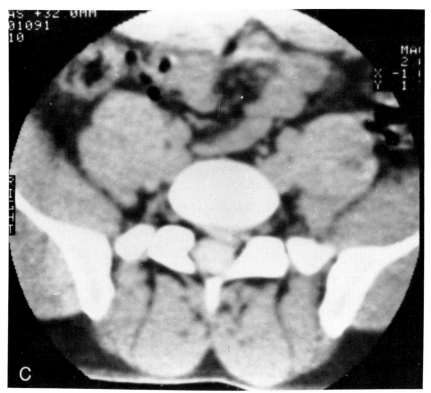

Figure 9.1. *C*, CT scan showing an HNP protruding into this insensitive space.

burning or temperature changes. Back findings are limited, with loss of range of movement and spasm often absent.

The most striking feature in this group of patients is the better than expected straight leg raising and the marked neurological lesion. One might theorize that compression of the nerve root in the limited confines of the foramen would indeed cause significant neurological signs. But why does it not cause, at the same time, significant neurological tension and thus significant limitation of straight leg raising? Either something happens within the nerve to allow for better straight leg raising (unlikely) or straight leg raising reduction is due to something other than root tension, *i.e.*, root inflammation.

We believe the latter is the explanation. In spinal stenosis the SLR is not significantly limited. On myeloscopy we have noted that the stenosed nerve root is held firmly and does not move. In the usual posterolateral HNP the nerve root does move on SLR testing and pain with this maneuver pulls the root off the eminence of the ruptured disc, mechanically disturbing the inflammatory boundary between the nerve root and

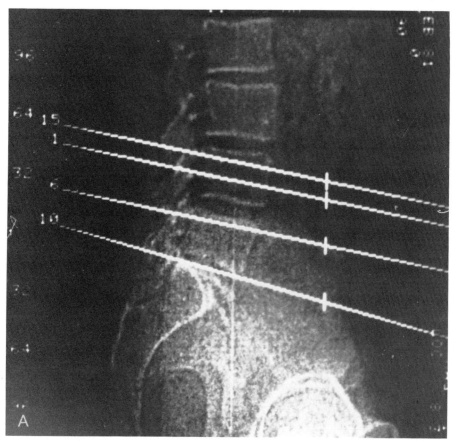

Figure 9.2. *A,* localizer film accompanying patient sent for chemonucleolysis.

the ruptured disc. Thus, a nerve root firmly held by a foraminal herniation does not manifest significant straight leg raising reduction.

The Midline Disc Herniation

The central disc herniation with bladder and bowel involvement is
recognized by all as a surgical emergency and is a contraindication to
chemonucleolysis. But, more and more disc herniations are now being
recognized with the CT scan as lying in the midline of the spinal canal
but not affecting bladder and bowel function (Fig. 9.5).

The patients are in the younger age group (25 to 40) as are those with
other disc herniations. Their dominant complaint is usually back pain
that may or may not have started with an injury. This history is usually
quite long because of the difficulty in recognizing the midline disc. With
the long history (years) is a story of remissions and exacerbations.

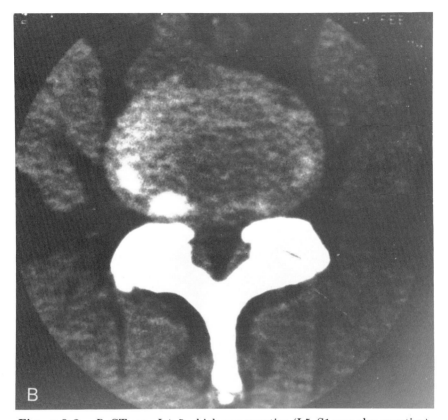

Figure 9.2. *B,* CT scan L4–5 which was negative (L5–S1 was also negative).

Both legs are affected, either together or more often alternating. If the disc herniation is a little more to one side than the other, that leg will tend to be more affected. The leg symptoms are quite variable and include classic sciatic distribution of pain, a deep sensation in the buttock only, calf cramps, especially at night when trying to fall sleep, and various symptoms, the most classic being paresthesia in the distribution of the involved nerve root.

On physical examination the patient will demonstrate decreased forward flexion with rigidity and flattening in the lumbar region on this movement. Yet backward extension is mobile and often normal because the dura is not being tented over the midline protrusion. At rest there is little muscle spasm.

Straight leg raising is reduced bilaterally and variably. The pain on straight leg raising is more often back pain but can be identical in location to the pain of straight leg raising in a classic disc herniation. The pathognomonic sign (infrequently present) is back and/or buttock discomfort on bowstring pressure in the popliteal fossa. Unlike an ex-

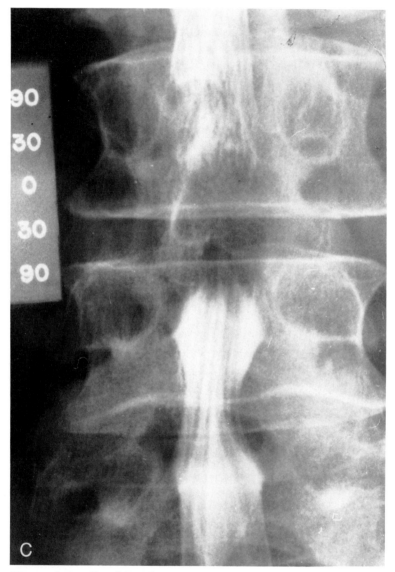

Figure 9.2. *C* and *D,* subsequent myelogram showing defect at L3–4.

treme lateral disc herniation, neurological signs are usually minimal. The CT scan is the important diagnostic test for midline HNP.

Although it is convenient to think of disc herniations or protrusions as being either classic in location, or extreme lateral or midline, it is not possible to clinically classify every patient in this manner. But common to all patients with back pain and sciatica due to nuclear protrusion (except midline) is the dominance of sciatica in a typical distribution,

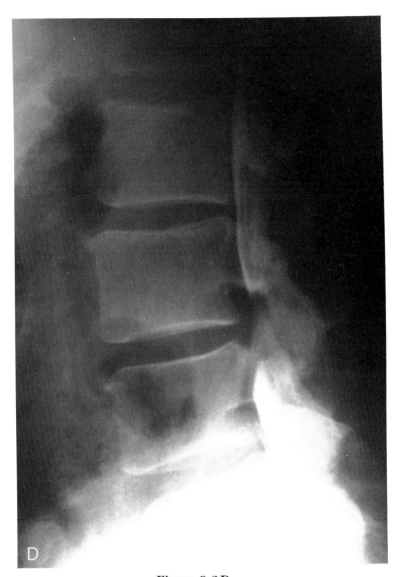

Figure 9.2D.

with neurological symptoms and/or signs and with pain on straight leg raising, indicating root tension or irritation.

Spinal Stenosis

Obviously spinal stenosis is not amenable to treatment by chemonucleolysis. But patients with spinal stenosis, that may or may not have been symptomatic, may report a sudden change in their status due to protrusion of nuclear material compromising an already narrow spinal

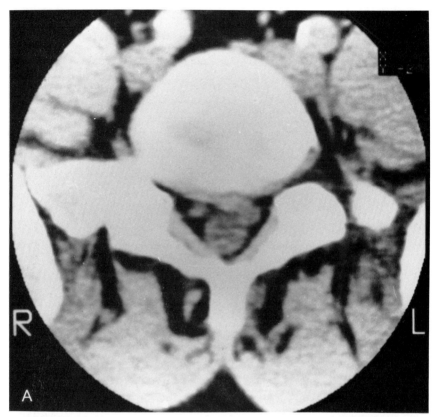

Figure 9.3. *A,* CT scan L5–S1 showing an HNP midline and left. Notice the apparent separation between the disc fragment and the posterior limits of the vertebral body/disc space, possibly indicating a sequestered disc. The patient has an excellent response to chemonucleolysis.

canal or lateral recess. The symptoms of these patients will then join the common thread of increasing leg pain, often unilateral, with a sudden change in neurological symptoms and/or signs and straight leg raising changes indicating increased root tension or irritation.

It has been impossible to make the diagnosis with conventional contrast investigations, but again CT scanning is coming to our rescue to help sort out bone from soft disc compression of the contents of the spinal canal (Fig. 9.6). However, the CT scan must be tempered with the clinical findings. Commonly the CT scan will show lateral recess stenosis at multiple levels, but the patient only demonstrates compromise of one root.

If you can identify the patient with spinal stenosis, who in addition has an associated clinical picture demonstrating that common thread of

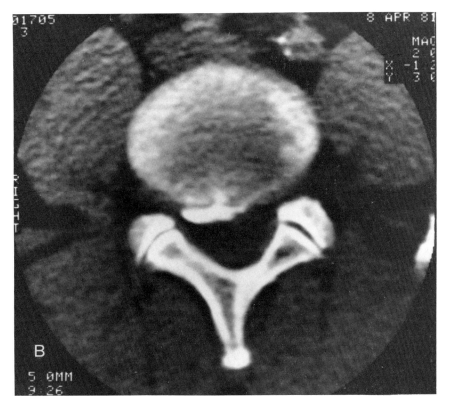

Figure 9.3. *B,* CT scan showing a calcified HNP—a contraindication to chemonucleolysis.

root tension, irritation, or compression, then you may improve the clinical state with chemonucleolysis. However, the use of chymopapain in the treatment of spinal stenosis by itself is useless.

OTHER CLINICAL PRESENTATIONS THAT MAY BE ENCOUNTERED

Postsurgery

The use of chymopapain will not resolve surgical failures. There is no point in attempting a chemonucleolysis in this patient (unless the previous operation was done at the wrong level or on the wrong side).

But a patient who has had previous successful surgery for a soft disc herniation with sciatica will sometimes (10%) experience recurrent symptoms suggesting a recurrent or new disc herniation. There must be a latent interval (usually months or years) between the successful surgery and the recurrent symptoms. The recurrent symptoms and signs still must have that thread of dominant leg pain, neurological symptoms and

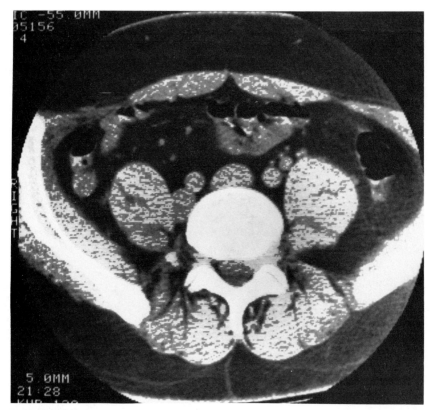

Figure 9.4. CT scan showing an HNP in foramen left at L5–S1. The myelogram was normal.

signs (changed and not residual), and straight leg raising changes indicative of root tension and irritation.

Venography is of no use in these patients. Myelography is of limited use if the disc herniation is at the same level and on the same side. Otherwise myelography is of value. So far, we do not think the CT scan is capable of distinguishing scar tissue from disc herniation tissue (Fig. 9.7). Probably the most significant investigative step is abolition of pain by nerve root infiltration with a local anesthetic.

Significant Neurological Changes

Occasionally a patient with a significant root lesion as measured by profound weakness will be seen. Usually, but not always, this patient will also have an absent reflex, an obvious sensory loss, and wasting. If the leg pain has largely resolved and straight leg raising is normal, there is no evidence that chemonucleolysis will improve the neurological lesion any quicker than letting nature take its course. If the neurological lesion

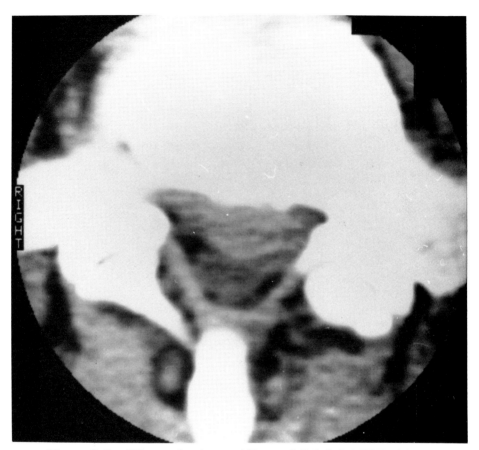

Figure 9.5.   CT scan showing a midline and slightly left HNP, L5–S1.

is accompanied by resolving pain and improving straight leg raising, then
again natural means should prevail. If the profound neurological lesion
is associated with persistent sciatica and a normal degree of straight leg
raising, then consider an extreme lateral disc herniation and seek CT
scan verification before considering chemonucleolysis. If the profound
neurological lesion is associated with significant straight leg raising
limitation due to pain, yet the complaint of sciatica is resolving, chemonucleolysis is indicated (provided the patient has pursued adequate
conservative care). A disc rupture, with profound neurological changes,
reduced SLR, and continuing sciatica as a symptom, is also an indication
for chemonucleolysis. Although the brochure accompanying Discase
states to the contrary, the authors feel that a severely compromised nerve
root is better decompressed by chymopapain thus avoiding the surgical
trauma and manipulation of an open approach. The one exception to

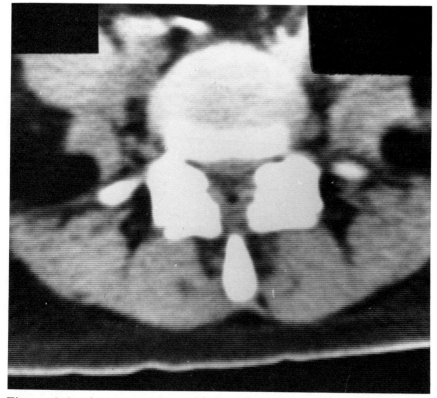

Figure 9.6. A young patient with lateral recess stenosis and some canal stenosis, with a midline HNP, L5–S1.

this is the association of a very large myelographic defect, with part of the defect away from the disc space, suggesting a sequestered disc. We are concerned that the injection of test material and 2 ml of chymopapain will add further volume compression to an already severely compromised nerve root, worsening the neurological situation.

A profound neurological deficit, in the absence of sciatica or any root tension and irritation, may be due to an intrathecal or extradural tumor. Investigation will reveal the mass.

Finally, patients with bladder and bowel involvement due to a nuclear herniation (usually sequestration) do not need any more volume compromise of their spinal canal and thus chemonucleolysis is contraindicated. The neurological root lesion that progresses quickly to a profound state should probably be decompressed surgically. Table 9.1 summarizes these concepts.

Remember, in considering a patient for chemonucleolysis, you are a pain doctor. Look for that common thread of root tension, irritation, and compression. In the face of a profound neurological lesion and the absence of that thread, the problem may be purely neurological, such as a tumor

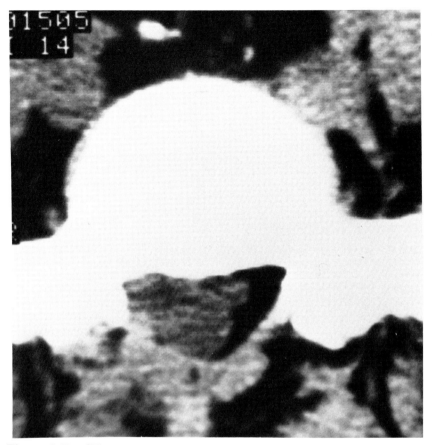

Figure 9.7.   CT scan in a postoperative patient with recurrent right leg pain. Is the defect scar or nuclear material?

or amyotrophic lateral sclerosis, etc., unrelated to abnormal movement of disc material. Do not consider chemonucleolysis.

Age

The average age of a patient with a disc herniation is 40 years. That does not mean that a person 70 years of age cannot have a disc herniation. It is less likely that patients in this age group will have back symptoms because of a disc rupture, but if they have that common thread of dominant leg pain, reduced straight leg raising, crossover pain, or a positive bowstring test, with neurological symptoms or signs, then this may very well be an older patient with a herniated nucleus pulposus who would respond to chemonucleolysis. In our center we recently had an 80-year-old woman complete a marathon run before many half her age. Anything is possible and just because the patient is old does not mean he does not have a disc herniation.

Table 9.1.

Lesion Neurological	Leg Pain	SLR	Preferred Treatment
Significant root (after sciatic pain improved)	None	Normal	Conservative
Significant root	Improving	Improving	Conservative
Significant root	Worsening	Decreased	Surgical or discolysis decompression
Significant root	Persistent	Slight decrease	Consider lateral disc herniation and then chemonucleolysis
Significant root	Improving	Persistent; significant decrease	Chemonucleolysis indicated
Significant root	Persistent	Persistent decrease	Chemonucleolysis indicated
Significant root	Persistent	Persistent decrease	In face of large myelographic defect, consider surgical decompression because of high incidence of sequestered disc and risk of worsening neurological status
Significant root	Absent or minimal	Normal	Consider tumor or other neurological conditions
Bladder and bowel involvement	Present in any degree	Any degree of reduction	Surgical decompression

The adolescent may fall victim to an HNP, which in our experience has responded well to chemonucleolysis. Our youngest patient has been 13 years. Because a disc herniation in adolescents tends not to be sequestered (5), they are ideal candidates for chymopapain injection.

Duration of Symptoms

There is no agreement between the authors on the significance of prolonged symptoms. The longer the back disability has been present, the more likely other degenerative changes will supersede the disc herniation and the patient's symptoms will not be amendable to treatment with chymopapain. But if a patient with prolonged symptoms is seen with that common thread of dominant leg pain, neurological symptoms and/or signs accompanied by significant root tension and irritation, then he may have a soft disc herniation that will respond to chemonucleolysis. The chance of a good response in this situation increases when the prolonged history has been associated with remissions and exacerbations and decreases when this history is one of persistent symptoms.

Nonorganic Factors

As mentioned in Chapter 7 on pain and disability, the presence of nonorganic reactions does not immunize the patient against a disc herniation. In the presence of nonorganic reaction, the common thread of root tension, root irritation, and root compression must be present and must be supported by irrefutable investigative evidence.

CONSERVATIVE CARE

Before considering chemonucleolysis, patients with sciatica due to a herniated lumbar disc *must* have adequate conservative care. Adequate conservative care is defined as not less than 2 weeks of complete bed rest or not less than 3 months of ambulatory care with avoidence of aggravating work and leisure activity, back support in a brace or corset, and supportive pain, anti-inflammatory and muscle relaxant medication.

Nonoperative care fails in one of three ways: 1) sciatica persists in spite of bed rest; 2) sciatica recurs after adequate bed rest; or 3) the neurological lesion increases in severity during bed rest.

The parameters used to evaluate response to conservative treatment are: duration of symptoms; degree of discomfort/degree of SLR reduction; degree of neurological involvement; and recurrence of symptoms after good conservative care.

Duration of Symptoms

Providing a severe neurological root lesion is not present, there are very few patients who should undergo chemonucleolysis within a few weeks of onset of symptoms. The majority of patients with sciatica will improve with adequate conservative care. It is unusual for a patient to undergo chemonucleolysis before 6 weeks has passed from the onset of symptoms, and preferably 3 months of care should occur. Severe sciatica or advancing neurological deficit will, on occasion, force a physician to intervene sooner.

Degree of Discomfort and the Degree of Straight Leg Raising Reduction

If, with adequate rest or ambulatory care, sciatic discomfort does not decrease, then the patient is a candidate for chemonucleolysis. The degree of discomfort should be assessed along with straight leg raising improvement. If both remain unchanged after acceptable conservative care, then the patient should be considered for chemonucleolysis.

If one improves without the other (usually the complaint of sciatica improves before straight leg raising), then persistent conservative care is in order. Sometimes the patient will reach a point of reasonable comfort with limited activity, but each time activity is increased (*e.g.*, returning to work) sciatica recurs. Root tension will persist as shown by marked limitation of SLR. Such a patient is a candidate for chemonucleolysis.

Degree of Neurological Involvement

Neurological symptoms, and/or signs, unaccompanied by root tension (SLR reduction) are not an indication for chemonucleolysis. Neurological symptoms and signs are the last to recover after root tension and irritation have subsided. If root tension and irritation subside with good conservative care, do not intervene with chemonucleolysis: the residual neurological symptoms and signs will probably improve spontaneously, albeit slowly.

Recurrence of Symptoms After Good Conservative Care

Not infrequently, good conservative care will lead to improvement in symptoms only to have them recur when ambulation begins. Symptoms may not recur for months or years after successful conservative care. The more frequent the recurrences, the closer they occur as episodes, the longer the episode lasts, and the greater the interference with patterns of living, the more indication there is for chemonucleolysis. On a rare occasion a patient from a remote area will be seen with acute sciatica and we are inclined to consider chemonucleolysis. A recent example was a missionary from South America who was anxious to return to her charge but was concerned that her remote location would not allow for follow-up care to failed conservative treatment. She underwent a successful chemonucleolysis and is now back to her calling with little fear of recurrence of symptoms.

In spite of the best indications and the most rigid parameters of conservative care, there will still be the patient in whom adequate conservative care is not possible. This most often occurs in the young professional, just starting solo practice after years of training and mounds of debt who suddenly becomes disabled because of sciatica. You should still aim for adequate conservative care parameters, but sometimes it is difficult and it becomes necessary to consider chemonucleolysis earlier in such patients. One of the drawbacks to the innocuous CT scan is that these people, by dint of profession or association, have an early CT scan (within days of the onset of symptoms) adding more pressure to the treating surgeon. Adequate conservative care still remains the standard of treatment in these situations.

To summarize and stress: chemonucleolysis is the last step in conservative care before considering surgical intervention.

CONTRAINDICATIONS

The product brochure states that chymopapain injection is contraindicated in the following situations:

Situation	Reason
1. Known allergy to chymopapain	Significant risk of anaphylaxis
2. Previous injection of chymopapain	Increased risk of anaphylaxis
3. Neurological lesions of cord, *e.g.*, multiple sclerosis	Fear of aggravation of disorders of uncertain etiology
4. Bladder or bowel involvement in central disc	Additional volume of test material or chymopapain may further impair, on a

	permanent basis, bladder and bowel function
5. Pregnant women	Effect of chymopapain or by-products of disc dissolution on fetus are unknown
6. Adolescent	See discussion
7. Disc lesions in the spinal canal at cord levels	Effect of chymopapain at cord levels has not been studied in enough detail

Except for an adolescent with an HNP, we recommend following the dictates of the product brochure.

Major Contraindication

The most important contraindication to chemonucleolysis is the absence of sciatica. Chymopapain will not assist in the management of degenerative disc disease, facet joint disease, spinal stenosis, spondylolisthesis, or any other low back disorder that does not have as its basis a soft disc herniation.

Chemonucleolysis will not dissolve away the problem of an emotional cripple.

Chemonucleolysis must never be performed because the surgeon is unwilling to carry out a laminectomy! This cannot be emphasized strongly enough.

Three specific situations that are not contraindications require comment.

SEQUESTERED DISC

To date the authors have no reliable clinical indicator of a sequestered disc. We are quick to agree that a free fragment of collagenous nuclear material in the spinal canal will not be affected by chymopapain. Unfortunately, we have no clinical description of this condition. A younger patient, with the sudden onset of almost exlusively leg pain, with neurological impairment and a moderate myelographic defect is suspected of having a sequestered disc, but enough of these patients respond to chemonucleolysis that the procedure is not contraindicated in them. We have several patients with a myelographic defect behind the vertebral body. Obviously they have a free fragment in the canal and this represents a contraindication to chemonucleolysis.

However, on most occasions there are only two ways to verify that a sequestered disc exists. First, operate on the patient and observe directly the pathology. Secondly, do chemonucleolysis and, if the procedure fails because of persisting sciatica, there is a 50% chance the patient has a sequestered disc.

There is a hope that as CT scanning software improves, the sequestered disc will be demonstrated and spare the patient the fruitless step of chemonucleolysis.

Leak of Test Material into the Epidural Space at the Time of Discometry (Discography) (Fig. 9.8)

Frequently test material will leak into the extradural space at the time of discometry or discography. This is not a contraindication to chemo-

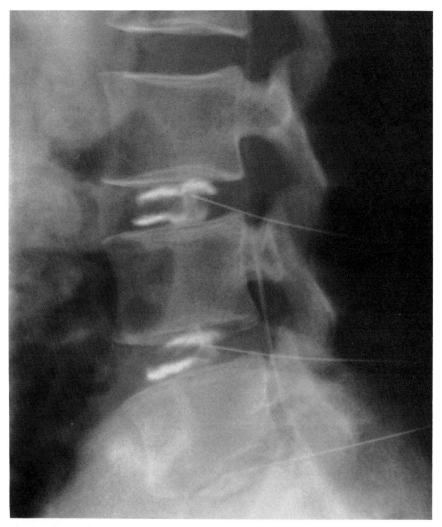

Figure 9.8. Leak of contrast material into the epidural space at the time of discography, L5–S1. This is not a contraindication to chemonucleolysis.

nucleolysis—it is the authors' opinion that there is no adverse reaction to chymopapain in the extradural space, borne out by extensive clinical and experimental experience.

Significant Root Neurological Lesion

An advancing or significant root lesion is not a contraindication to chymopapain decompression. In fact, it seems more sensible to decompress the compromised nervous tissue with the least manipulation possible, *i.e.*, chemonucleolysis rather than surgical decompression. We are leaning away from chemonucleolysis when a significant neurological lesion is accompanied by a large myelographic defect (Table 9.1).

Why Do Chemonucleolysis? Why Not Surgical Laminectomy, Discectomy?

It is natural for a surgeon to prefer a surgical solution for a mass lesion in the spinal canal. He can view the pathology, he can remove a sequestered disc, and he can handle other pathology such as lateral recess stenosis. Why should you consider a percutaneous closed procedure to remove a herniated disc?

You should consider this method of treatment as the last step in conservative treatment for the following reasons:

1. The procedure is simple and safe for the patient. There is little downside risk to the patient and its simplicity for patient and surgeon, when compared to laminectomy, is striking.
2. The procedure is effective in relieving sciatica in 70% of properly selected patients. Adhering to the criteria described in this chapter, you can confidently expect a high rate of success.
3. Demands on health care facilities are reduced dramatically by use of chemonucleolysis rather than laminectomy and discectomy (6).
4. For the patient pressed for time, chemonucleolysis may offer a shortcut back to gainful employment. The authors have reduced total time required for investigation and treatment in some instances down to one day. We have experienced stoic patients who return to work the day after chemonucleolysis. This does not appear to be detrimental to a good result, but at the same time it is not recommended as optimal postinjection care. However, when the patient's circumstances are such that he requests this care, it is a consideration you can entertain as a surgeon.
5. Epidural scarring is a natural sequel to open surgery and the entrance of blood into the laminotomy defect and extradural space. Scarring postsurgery is minimal in some patients but a serious detriment to a good result in many patients. Scarring as a complication is not even a consideration in chemonucleolysis.
6. There are no bridges burned with chemonucleolysis. If the procedure is not successful in relieving the patient's symptoms, surgical consideration can be made without any concern for untoward effects of the prior chemonucleolysis.
7. It is the authors' experience and theoretically acceptable to state that successful chemonucleolysis will offer the patient a long-term good result. Chymopapain will remove all nuclear material to the point where recurrence is very unusual. The absence of a midline ligamentous and muscular detachment exposure and the absence of an opening into the extradural space preserve natural tissue support in the region and reduce long-term mechanical and scarring complications directly attributable to open surgery.

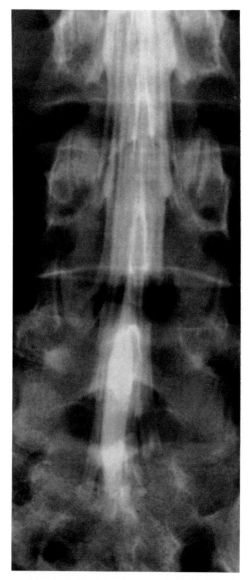

Figure 9.9. A double disc herniation, L4–5 one side, and L5–S1 opposite side.

There are many reasons to recommend chemonucleolysis rather than surgery when conservative care fails to relieve sciatica due to a soft disc herniation.

One Level or Two Level Injections

One topic that raises much controversy among users is whether one or multiple levels should be injected. The controversy is easily settled by stating that most patients should undergo single level injection of chymopapain. The reasoning is simple.

No patient for whom you do not confidently expect a good result to simple laminectomy and discectomy should undergo chemonucleolysis. These patients, with a disc herniation as the cause of sciatica, have single level pathology. We are sure your past surgical considerations have been largely single level for the simple disc herniation, and thus the chymopapain injection should be confined to a single level.

There are occasions when the basis of your surgical decision erodes as you enter the interlaminar space to discover little in the way of pathology. You might then explore a second level but if this is your surgical routine for sciatica due to a soft disc herniation, you are not preselecting your patients or your level of exploration well enough. We are all entitled to the occasional miss, and the requirement for a two level surgical exploration, and similarly we are entitled to an occasional insecure diagnosis and a two level chemonucleolysis. However, if this becomes your routine, you are not selecting your patients well. Other reasons for two level injections are the infrequent double disc herniation (Fig. 9.9) and the postsurgical patient with a disc herniation at a new level and persistent symptoms arising from the previous surgical level. These situations are so infrequent that you cannot escape the thrust that, just as most disc herniations causing sciatica occur at single levels, so should most chymopapain injections be confined to a single level.

References

1. McCulloch JA: Chemonucleolysis. *J Bone Joint Surg* 59:45, 1977.
2. McCulloch JA: Chemonucleolysis. Experience with 2000 cases. *Clin Orthop* 146:128, 1980.
3. Postacchini F: Extreme lateral herniations of lumbar discs. *Clin Orthop* 138:222, 1979.
4. Abdullah AF, Ditto EW, Byrd EB, *et al.*: Extreme lateral lumbar disc herniations. *J Neurosurg* 41:229, 1974.
5. Kurihara A, Katoaka O: Lumbar disc herniation in children and adolescents. *Spine* 5:443, 1980.
6. McCulloch JA, Ferguson JM: Outpatient chemonucleolysis. *Spine* 6:606, 1981.

CHAPTER **10**

Technique of Chemonucleolysis

Surgery is so simple! Know the correct indications, pick the right patient, then do the procedure properly. This chapter is concerned with the technique of chemonucleolysis which, once learned, is also simple. Before the authors arrived at a point of making chemonucleolysis a simple procedure, we made a number of mistakes and learned new concepts. These we share with you.

BASIC CONSIDERATIONS

Chemonucleolysis, chemical excision of nucleus pulposus, is an operation. It requires the skill of an individual capable of recognizing the patient who will benefit from the procedure, capable of looking after immediate or delayed complications, and capable of intervening surgically in those patients who fail to respond. We do not recommend the procedure be divided up among a number of specialty areas, but rather one person should be facile in all aspects of diagnosis and treatment so that all the benefits and pitfalls of the procedure can be grasped.

Chemonucleolysis must be done in a hospital setting, using sterile technique. The best setting is an operating room and second best is a radiology department. We have had a long string of successes with clean discography because of our operating room setting, sterile technique, and in particular "no touch" technique. Figure 10.1 depicts the tray we use. During "no touch," we try not to handle the shaft of any needle or the inner workings of any syringe.

Do not attempt the procedure without an anesthesiologist who is capable of handling the acute emergency of anaphylaxis. To do otherwise courts disaster. For the same reason do not start the procedure without an intravenous setup with a large bore catheter in place.

Two areas of controversy require addressing:
1. Is this procedure done on an inpatient or outpatient basis?
2. Is this procedure done under local or general anesthesia?

Our preference is to perform this procedure on an outpatient basis whenever possible and to use a local anesthetic.

OUTPATIENT CHEMONUCLEOLYSIS

The objection to this type of hospital setting has been the significant back pain some patients have after chemonucleolysis. Pain does occur in a few patients, requiring hospitalization of patients from the outpatient department, but 98% of our patients selected for outpatient chemonucleolysis manage without overnight hospital admission. Some of them have significant back pain or spasms afterwards but, forewarned of the nature and management, cope well with the situation.

Appendix I is an outline of instructions given to patients before the

128

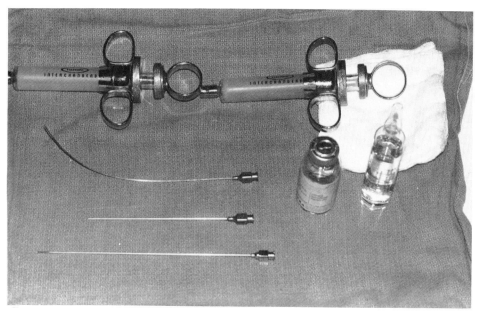

Figure 10.1. Tray setup with two syringes: needles (*top to bottom*) are: 6-inch 22-gauge with curve, 4-inch 18-gauge, and 6-inch 18-gauge; local anesthetic; sterile water for injection (USP) for: a)reconstitution of chymopapain and b) discometry.

procedure. This allays many fears and helps immensely in the management of patients, especially on an outpatient basis. Patients in the older age group or patients with medical problems are managed as inpatients. Fortunately, most sufferers of herniated nucleus pulposus (HNP) are young and healthy and thus chemonucleolysis can be done on an outpatient basis.

GENERAL ANESTHESIA OR LOCAL ANESTHESIA

The two decades of clinical experience with chemonucleolysis have left the controversy of anesthesia for this procedure unresolved. Those supporting general anesthesia cite the following reasons:

1. The complication of anaphylaxis requires general anesthesia and intubation for control.
2. The procedure is too painful for patients to experience without general anesthesia.

Those who support local anesthesia cite the following reasons:

1. The complication of anaphylaxis is best managed without the complication of a general anesthetic. Awake, the patient has an early warning system working. The sensation of burning, tingling, coldness, nausea, and vomiting may precede the reaction by minutes and allow early treatment of anaphylaxis. If the blood pressure is not being taken

every minute under general anesthetic, the early stages of anaphylaxis where treatment is most effective will be missed. In fact, we now routinely abort anaphylactic reactions using this early warning system and aggressive management (*cf.* Chapter 12, Adverse Reactions to Chymopapain).

2. Respiratory distress is not a consideration when anaphylaxis is managed early and aggressively. We have witnessed 15 anaphylactic reactions in patients under local anesthesia without one patient requiring intubation (*cf.* Chapter 12, Adverse Reactions to Chymopapain).

3. There are specific contraindications to the combination of the general anesthetic agent, fluothane, and adrenaline (2).

4. The procedure is not particularly hard on the patient under local anesthesia.

5. The value of discography is such that it should not be given up to general anesthesia (*cf.* Chapter 10, section on discometry).

6. Some patients, under general anesthesia in other centers, were the victims of penetration of the fifth lumbar root as it emerged from the foramen. Some subsequently developed a fifth root palsy. Awake, the patients will not allow penetration of any nerve root. It is very painful!

7. Finally, the use of this procedure on an outpatient basis is facilitated by local anesthesia.

In summary, our recommendation is for local anesthesia with neuroleptic augmentation and not general anesthesia with intubation.

OUR LOCAL NEUROLEPTIC ANESTHETIC ROUTINE

1. The patient receives no premedication.

2. An intravenous infusion with a large bore catheter is started in the operating room.

3. Intravenous diazepam and fentanyl, in appropriate doses, are given.

4. Needle insertion is carried out using local anesthesia.

5. Discography (discometry) is carried out.

6. Before chymopapain is injected, a low dose of Sodium Pentothal is injected IV to take the patient to a drowsy state of anesthesia but allow for the patient to return to a conscious state within a moment of injection of the chymopapain.

THE OPERATING ROOM

In some centers this procedure is carried out in the x-ray department. We recommend that the procedure be done in the operating room where members of the anesthesia staff, nursing staff, and recovery room staff are well skilled in the handling of urgent situations such as anaphylaxis. Most x-ray departments and staff, although equipped to handle such an emergency, have not had the depth of experience of an operating room staff in coping with these events. A problem occurs when the best equipment for doing the procedure is in the x-ray department, and the best group of personnel for managing the complications is the in operating room. We suggest you upgrade you operating room x-ray equipment so

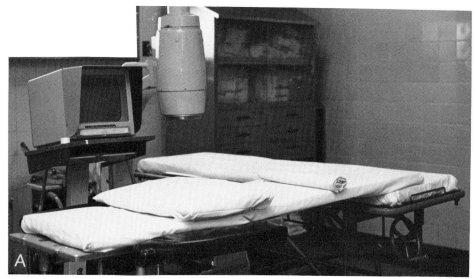

Figure 10.2. *A,* operating room setup: simply a piece of 1-inch plywood, placed between an operating table and a stretcher.

that the procedure can be done there. Figure 10.2 depicts our operating room setup.

THE LATERAL APPROACH

Because chymopapain will cause dissolution of the basement membranes of blood vessels in the subarachnoid space, the procedure must be done using the posterolateral discographic approach. Crossing the spinal canal with a needle, through which chymopapain will be injected, risks leakage of chymopapain into the subarachnoid space which may cause fatal subarachnoid hemorrhage.

This approach was first described by Lindblom (3) and was the basis for our paper (4) and this chapter.

It makes little difference if the lateral approach is carried out from the right or the left. For the purpose of this chapter, assume that the patient is lying on the left side and the approach is from the right side.

In trying to grasp the intricacies of this procedure, think of approaching the patient in six phases:
1. Maintain proper positioning of the patient.
2. Select the correct disc.
3. Select the correct needle insertion site.
4. Approach the disc at the proper angle.
5. Position the needle tip in the middle of the disc.
6. Appreciate all the intricacies of discometry (discography).
7. Inject the proper amount of active chymopapain into a clean disc space.

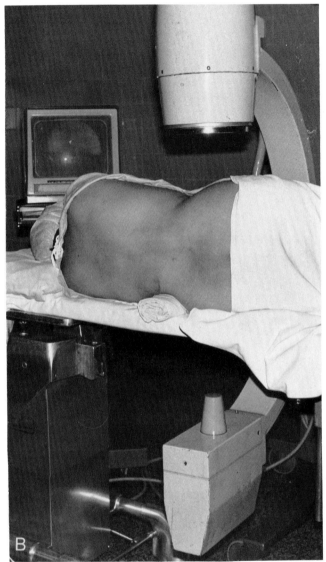

Figure 10.2.   *B*, patient in position and a C-arm image intensifier set up for lateral image.

Maintain Proper Positioning of the Patient

With patients under local neuroleptic anesthesia and in the lateral decubitus position, it is very easy for them to roll out of position and introduce an oblique dimension to a difficult problem, *i.e.*, the three-dimensional problem of getting a needle into the disc space using the two-dimensional aid in the form of an image intensifier.

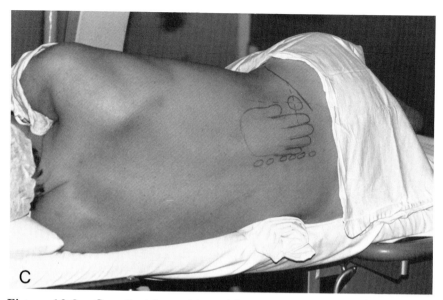

Figure 10.2. *C,* patient in position with spinous processes, iliac crest, and "hand's breadth" marked. Note rolled sheet under flank to reduce scoliosis.

The basic rule is to accept nothing less than a perfect lateral and anteroposterior image on the image intensifier screen. It is so easy to become engrossed in the problem of the needle entering the disc that you forget you have a patient, who may have rolled out of position.

Mistakes that you can make in regard to position are, in order of commission:

i. The patient rolls away from your probing with the needle, thereby introducing an oblique dimension (Fig. 10.3).
ii. The patient naturally pushes back with the head and shoulders and rolls away with the pelvis, the so-called corkscrew (Fig. 10.4).
iii. The patient arches the back into a scoliosis position through muscle tension.
iv. The patient arches the back into lordosis by straightening the legs. Always keep the legs in a 90:90 hip-knee positon (Fig. 10.5).
v. The patient's shoulders are so broad and the pelvis so narrow that positioning in the standard manner leaves the spine running downhill.
vi. The patient is positioned too close to the edge of the table and has to assume an oblique position to prevent rolling over the edge and onto the floor.

We have often stated that the three most important things to remember in trying to get a needle into a disc space are: position, position, and position. If you are having trouble, think of these three things. If you find the exercise particularly difficult, then there are tables and outrigger aids you may seek (5).

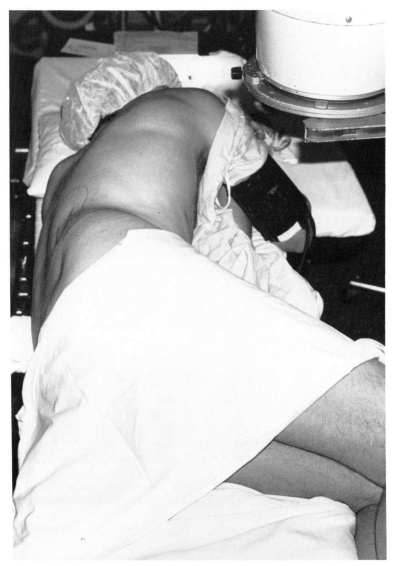

Figure 10.3. Patient has rolled shoulders away from surgeon, introducing an oblique dimension on the lateral x-ray.

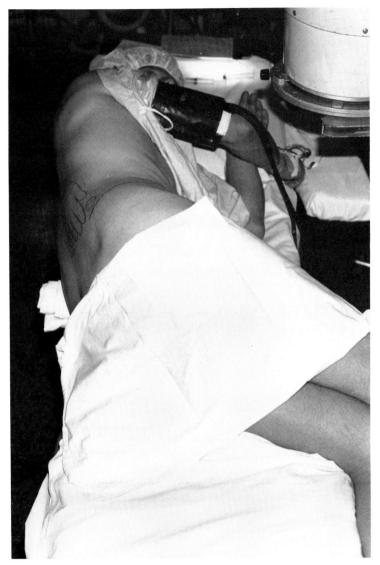

Figure 10.4. The "corkscrew" position, in which the patient pushes the shoulders back and rolls the hips forward. This also creates an oblique dimension to the lateral x-ray on the image intensifier screen.

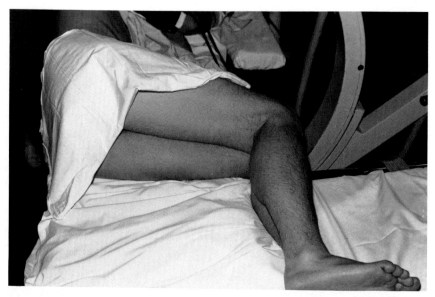

Figure 10.5. It is important to keep the hips and knees in a 90°:90° position to flatten the lumbar lordosis.

We make a habit of only prepping and draping the patient after the patient is positioned in the perfect lateral position, confirmed by the image intensifier. If the perfect lateral image disappears during the procedure, it is the patient who has moved, not the image intensifier. It is a fact that needs to be impressed on the overzealous x-ray technician who wants to move the image intensifier each time the patient moves; a cat and mouse situation that will have you, the surgeon, going around in circles.

Select the Correct Disc Space for Entry and Injection

This seems so basic that you probably find the statement insulting. Before your chemonucleolysis career is over, you will put the needle in the wrong disc space! We have done it, and fortunately recognized it, but to save you the embarassment we suggest the following two steps before you select the disc space:

KNOW WHICH DISC SPACE YOU ARE GOING TO INJECT BEFORE YOU START

It goes without saying that chymopapain will only be useful if injected into the correct disc. But it is so easy, with a limited image intensifier field and blinders on as to neurological involvement, to make the mistake of injecting the wrong disc space.

The patient presenting with sciatica-like symptoms is taken through the following steps:

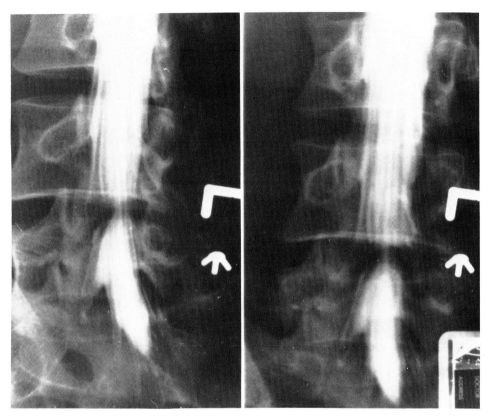

Figure 10.6. Patient with an HNP, L4-5 right, who was seen with S1 symptoms and signs. Note the right S1 root under tension from the HNP.

a. Is it sciatica? (*cf.* Chapters 5 and 9.)
b. If it is sciatica, what nerve root is involved? (*cf.* Chapters 5 and 9.)
c. When the nerve root involved has been identified, which disc space harbors the HNP? It is so easy to assume that S1 nerve root involvement means an L5-S1 HNP. But read on.

Wrong Level Disc Herniation

Most patients with a disc prolapse at L4-5 will have fifth root symptoms and signs, and most patients with fifth root symptoms and signs will have a disc prolapse at L4-5. Figures 10.6, 10.7, and 10.8 show exceptions and demonstrate that a disc herniation at one level has the potential of compromising three different roots depending on its direction of displacement, *e.g.*, an L4-5 disc prolapse migrating

a. Superiorly—may get L4 root.
b. Medially—may get S1 root.
c. Laterally—may get L4 root (foraminal), in addition to the common L5 root.

This concept is represented schematically in Figure 10.9.

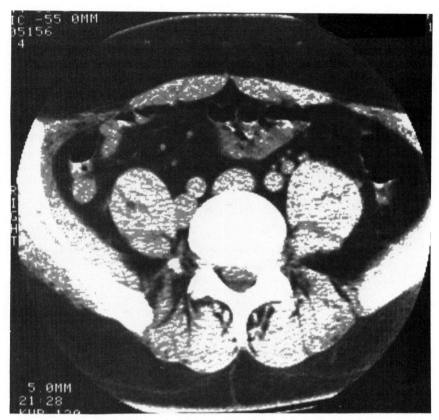

Figure 10.7. Foraminal HNP, L5-S1 left, with fifth root neurological symptoms and signs.

Congenital Lumbosacral Anomalies

Be aware of congenital lumbosacral anomalies and the traps that your radiological colleagues may have built for you by reporting disc herniations at L4-S1, L5-L6, and L4-L5 with six lumbar vertebrae.

We would strongly suggest that terminology used to describe normal lumbar spine anatomy be confined to those patients with normal lumbar spinal anatomy, *i.e.*, five lumbar vertebrae free of rib attachment and free of pelvic or sacral attachment. We further suggest that terminology L4-S1 and L5-L6 not be used when trying to describe abnormal lumbar spines. In fact, when there are an abnormal number of lumbar vertebrae or congenital lumbosacral anomalies, we should not use our standard terminology of L4-5 and L5-S1 and should not use the terms lumbarization and sacralization.

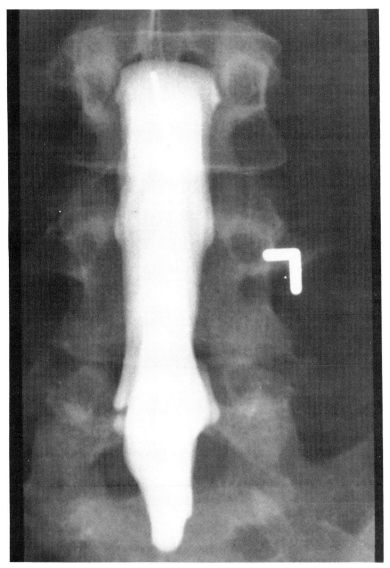

Figure 10.8. An HNP, L4-5 left, in a patient who was seen with anterior thigh pain and fourth lumbar root involvement. Part of the disc fragment had migrated superiorly to cause fourth root compression.

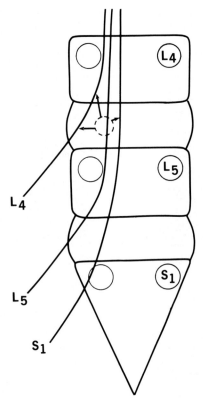

Figure 10.9. A disc herniation at L4-5 normally interferes with fifth root function. However, if it migrates laterally or superiorly it will impair the fourth root. If it migrates medially, it can impair first sacral root function (see Fig. 10.6).

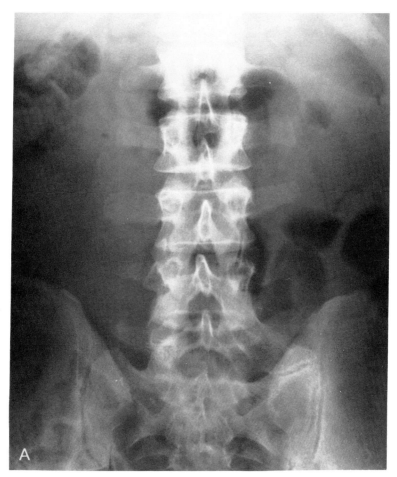

Figure 10.10. *A,* patient with six lumbar vertebrae with partial fixation of last formed lumbar segment on the left.

Figure 10.10 shows a patient with six lumbar levels without rib attachments, but the last lumbar level is attached to the pelvis. The radiologist reported the disc herniation at the L5-S1 level for reasons many would find acceptable. But imagine yourself with the patient in the lateral position with the image field as represented in Figure 10.11. Which level is L5-S1? Hopefully, you would not fall into the trap, but some have. Wouldn't it be much simpler (and safer) with any congenital lumbosacral anomaly to use the following terminology?
1. Last formed level (LFL)—a level with a separate spinous process, and/or an interlaminar space, and/or facet joints rudimentary or normal (Fig. 10.12).

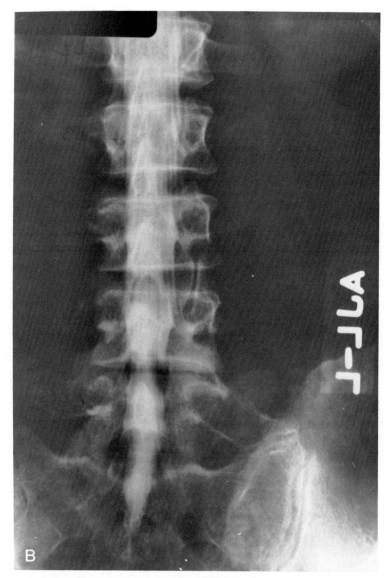

Figure 10.10. *B*, myelogram showing defect at last fully mobile level, and no defect at last formed lumbar level. It is immobile because of the fixation.

2. Last mobile level (LML)—a formed level free of any attachment to pelvis (Fig. 10.12).

In the normal skeleton, L5-S1 is the last formed level with posterior joints and an interlaminar space. It is also the last mobile level. But in Figure 10.11, the radiologist has numbered the second last formed level

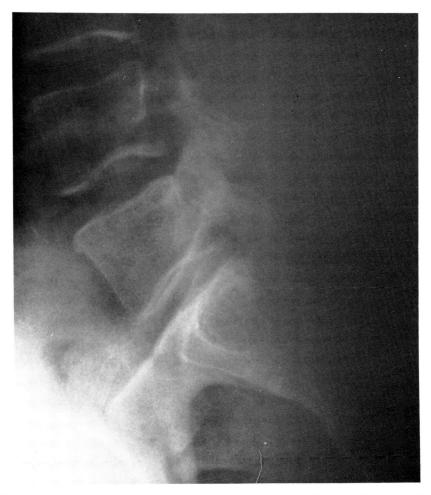

Figure 10.11.   Lateral view of lumbosacral region of patient in Figure 10.10.
The radiologist has reported the HNP at L5-S1.

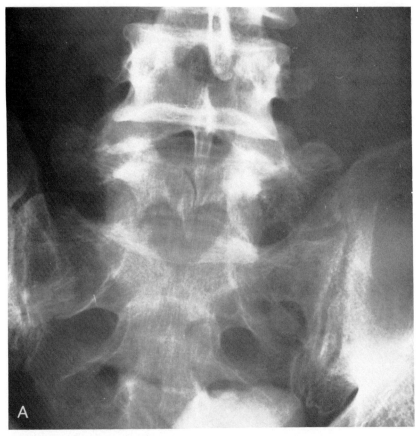

Figure 10.12. *A*, anteroposterior view of lumbosacral region showing the last formed level (LFL) with an interlaminar space, facet joints, and one transverse process free of pelvic attachment. The large transverse process on the opposite side, attached to the pelvis and sacrum, has probably removed all movement from the LFL. The level *above* thus becomes the last mobile level.

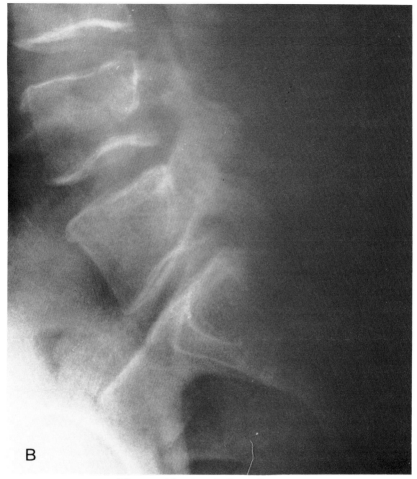

Figure 10.12.   *B*, lateral view.

(and last mobile level) as L5-S1, when it would have been safer to use the terminology 2LFL and LML.

Figures 10.13, 10.14, and 10.15 show more congenital lumbosacral anomalies with conventional and revised designations.

BE SURE TO SEE THE FRONT OF THE SACRUM BEFORE COUNTING

Look at Figure 10.16 and select L4-5. Now look at figure 10.17 and see which disc space you selected. Everyone learning to do chemonucleolysis invariably makes this mistake. The simple maneuver of moving the image intensifier down to the last formed level and seeing the front of the sacrum will keep you out of this trap.

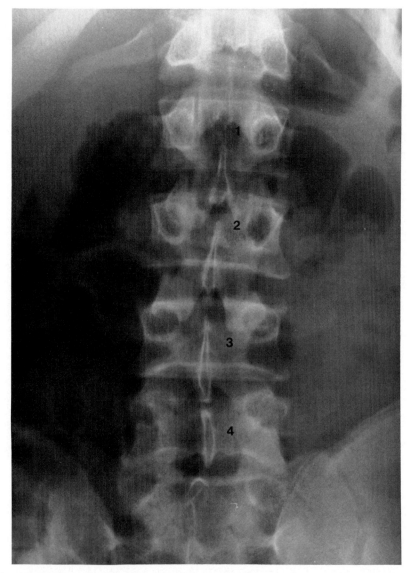

Figure 10.13. Four lumbar vertebrae, each free of pelvic attachment and rib formation. Below the fourth lumbar level, there are no facet joints or interlaminar space. Thus, the disc space between L4 and the sacrum is both the LFL and the LML.

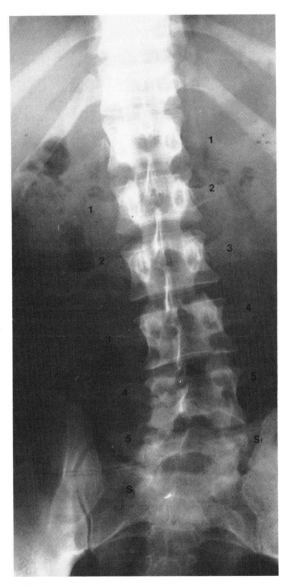

Figure 10.14. Four lumbar vertebrae, free of pelvic attachment and rib formation, which could be numbered in two different ways. Using the numbers on the left, the L5-S1 space is the LFL, and the level above (L4-5) is the LML.

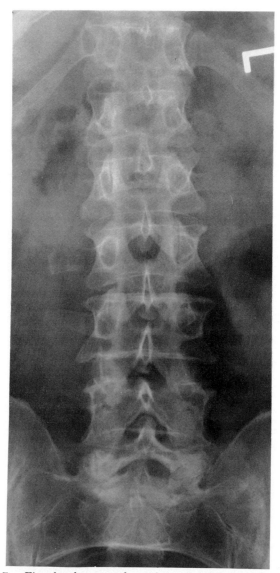

Figure 10.15. Five lumbar vertebrae free of pelvic attachment. However, there is a rudimentary level below, with an interlaminar space. Look closely at L1 where the transverse processes are actually short, rudimentary ribs. Thus, there are two ways to number the vertebrae on this x-ray, but no confusion if the terms "LFL" and "LML" are used.

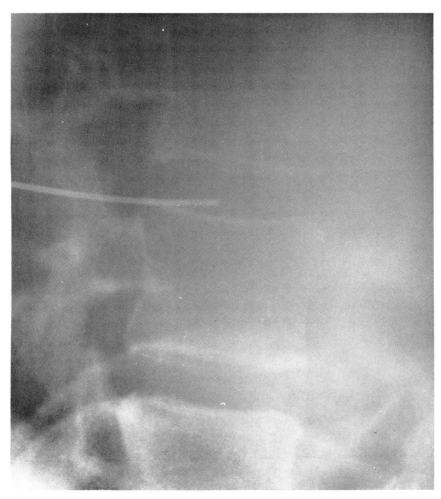

Figure 10.16. Needle thought to be in the L4-5 space.

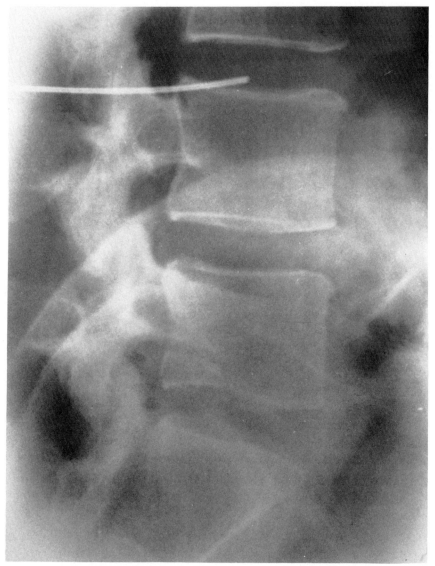

Figure 10.17.   Needle in L3-4. The front of the sacrum is clearly evident.

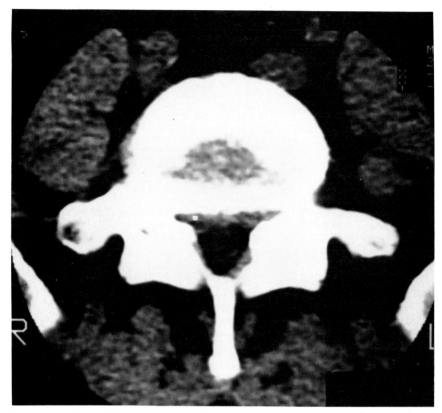

Figure 10.18. CT scan showing the anteroposterior orientation of the posterior elements: 1) pedicle and transverse process, most anteriorly; 2) facet joint, pars and lamina, intermediately; and 3) spinous process, most posteriorly.

Site of Insertion of the Needle and Angle of Approach to Disc Space

Figure 10.2C shows the selection of the site of insertion of the needle adjacent to the iliac crest and one hand's breadth from the midline.

As mentioned in the introduction, the technique of chemonucleolysis is carried out through the posterolateral approach. The skeletal structures most perplexing from this approach are the posterior elements. (It is fortunate that they are present to keep the needle out of the spinal canal and thus avoid the devastating complication of a subarachnoid injection.) Think of the posterior elements in the following manner.

LATERAL PROJECTION

From anterior to posterior, the elements are in three groups (Fig. 10.18): 1) pedicle and transverse process; 2) superior facet, pars interarticularis, inferior facet and lamina; and 3) spinous process.

You will appreciate this three-dimensional concept only by looking at a vertebral body.

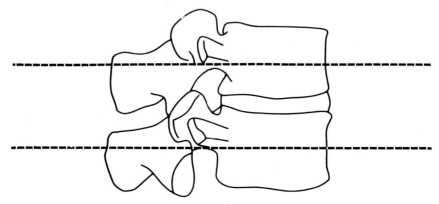

Figure 10.19. Lateral projection with imaginary line dividing vertebral body in half (see text for relevance).

ANTEROPOSTERIOR PROJECTION

In Figure 10.19, an imaginary line is drawn to divide the vertebral body in half. The posterior elements are now split into two groups:
1. Behind and superimposed on the superior half of the vertebral body lie the pedicle, transverse process, and superior facet.
2. Behind the posterior half lie the lamina, spinous process, and inferior facet. Joining the two groups is the pars interarticularis. Again, look at a vertebral segment to appreciate this.

Translating these posterior element anatomical relationships into technical consideration, you will note that:
a. Bony obstruction to needle advancement that occurs when the needle tip is level with the upper half of the vertebral body is usually due to the transverse process (Fig. 10.20).
b. Bony obstruction to needle advancement that occurs when the needle tip is level with the lower half of the vertebral body is usually due to the superior articular facet (Fig. 10.21).
c. Bony obstruction to needle advancement that occurs when the needle tip is level with the junction of the upper and lower halves is usually due to the pars interarticularis (Fig. 10.22).

Knowledge of these posterior element relationships will assist in needle placement within the nuclear area of the disc.

Approach the Disc at the Proper Angle

L4-5 DISC SPACE

The L4-5 disc space is approached first from a point at the level of the iliac crest and 10 cm (one hand's breadth) to the right of the midline (Fig. 10.23). The distance from the midline may be varied slightly to allow for the patient's build (*i.e.*, a little more lateral for big patients and a little more medial for small patients). If muscle spasm interferes with

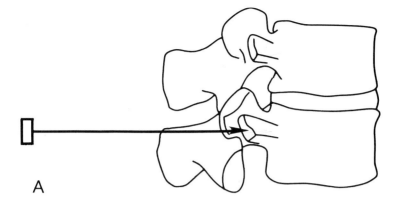

A

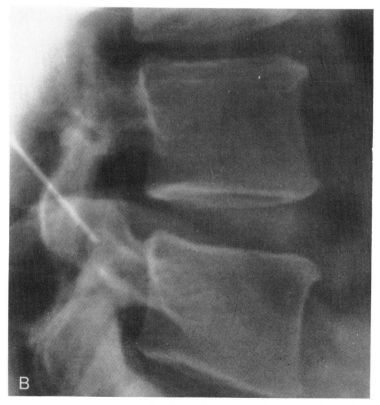

B

Figure 10.20. *A* and *B*, needle obstruction at level of upper half of vertebral body. Cause—transverse process.

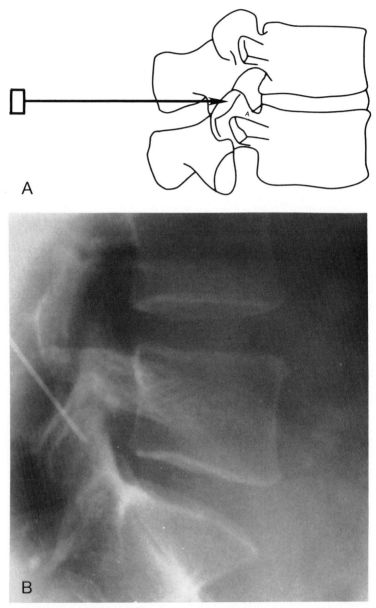

Figure 10.21.   *A* and *B*, needle obstruction at level of lower half of vertebral body. Cause—superior facet (of L5 in *A*; of S1 in *B*).

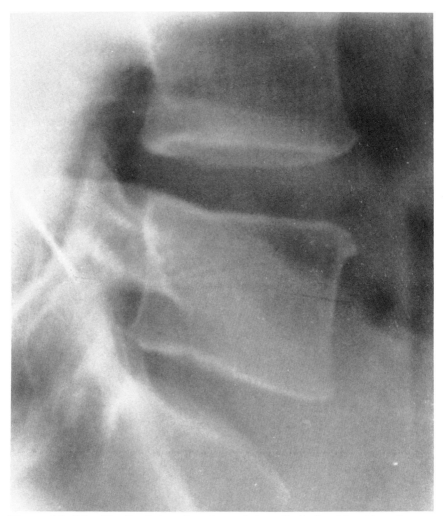

Figure 10.22. Needle obstruction at pars interarticularis, at junction of upper and lower halves of vertebral body.

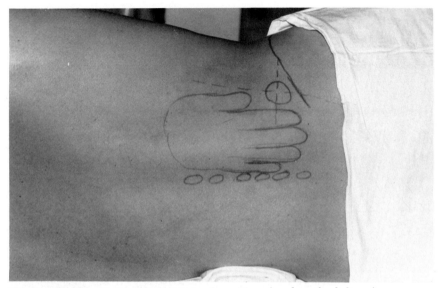

Figure 10.23. Patient in left lateral position, head to the left; spinous processes, iliac crest, and "one hand's breadth" marked.

localization of the spinous processes, the midline may be identified first in the lower thoracic region.

After superficial infiltration of local anesthetic, the 6-inch No. 18 needle is inserted at an angle of 50 to 60° to the sagittal plane in the direction of the L4-5 disc space. The lateral radiograph confirms that the needle is neither superior nor inferior to the disc space. If necessary, further local anesthetic may be infiltrated through the needle.

When the tip of the advancing needle reaches a line joining the posterior borders of the vertebral bodies, the surgeon should obtain a firm, gritty sensation from the annulus (Fig. 10.24). If the tip of the needle passes anterior to this line before this sensation is obtained (Fig. 10.25), the needle will not bisect the disc but will pass anterolateral to it. If this occurs, the angle of needle insertion is too close to 45° and should be changed nearer to 60° to the sagittal plane. When the angle is changed, the needle should first be withdrawn close to the skin surface.

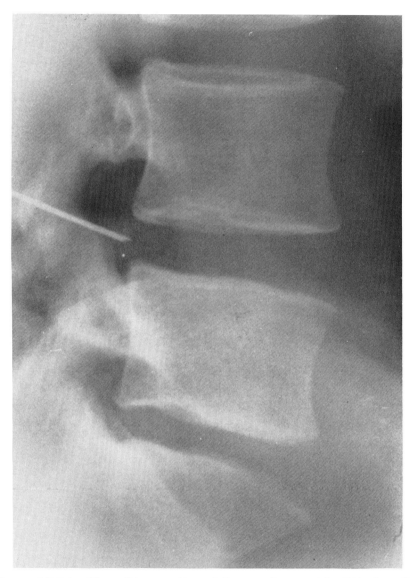

Figure 10.24. The gritty sensation of the annulus must be felt when the advancing needle tip reaches the imaginary line joining the posterior vertebral body margins (position *A*, in Fig. 10.26).

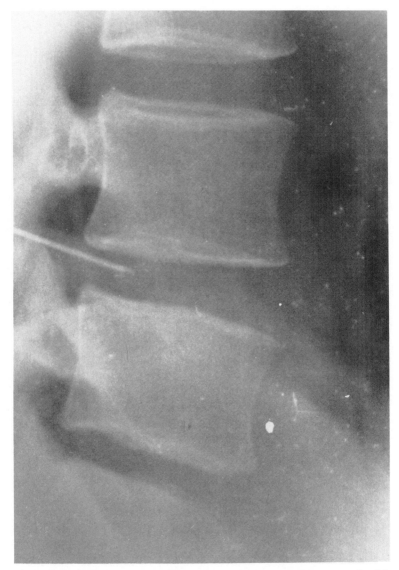

Figure 10.25. Needle tip in front of line joining posterior vertebral body margins, *without* the gritty feel of the annulus (position *B*, in Fig. 10.26).

Bony impingement at the level of the upper half of the vertebral body is probably due to the transverse process. Obstruction at the level of the lower half of the vertebral body is probably due to the tip of the superior facet. Opposite the disc space, obstruction is probably due to the lower portion of the facet joint. If the transverse process causes obstruction, the site of needle insertion is moved in a cephalad (for L4-5) or caudal (for L5-S1) direction. If the pars interarticularis or the facet joint causes obstruction, the angle of needle insertion needs to be reduced to below 60° from the sagittal plane. However, problems arise if too much attention is paid to the angle of needle insertion and too little to the overall size and shape of the patient. A clear, three-dimensional, mental image of the lower lumbar region is essential. An articulated specimen of the spine in the operating room is a helpful aid.

During the procedure, patients tend to rotate the pelvis away from the needle, introducing an oblique dimension to the lateral radiograph which will confuse the three-dimensional image and invalidate the technical details mentioned above. If difficulties do arise, it is advisable to pause, confirm that the patient remains in a truly lateral position, check the surface landmarks, and carefully scrutinize the overall anatomy.

When the annulus is successfully encountered, 0.5 to 1.0 ml of local anesthetic may be infiltrated (an unusual requirement) and the needle is advanced into the center of the disc. If the needle exactly bisects the disc, advancement of the needle by ½ inch should be accompanied by apparent advancement of approximately ¼ inch on lateral screening (Fig. 10.26A). If the needle passes across the lateral edge of the disc space, coming out anteriorly, advancement of the needle by ½ inch will be accompanied by close to ½ inch apparent advancement (Fig. 10.26B). Conversely, if the needle passes across the back of the disc space, a ½-inch advancement will be accompanied by very little apparent advancement on lateral x-ray (Fig. 10.26C). Once the needle is in the center of the disc space on the lateral view, the image intensifier is rotated to the anteroposterior view to confirm that the tip of the needle is in the midline. The needle tip must be medial to the pedicle.

L5-S1 DISC SPACE

The image intensifier is repositioned laterally. Local anesthetic is infiltrated ¼ inch medial and inferior to the L4-5 needle placement and a 4-inch No. 18 needle is inserted. The L4-5 needle serves as a landmark and guide to the position of the L5-S1 disc space. The L5-S1 needle is inserted at the same angle to the sagittal plane, *i.e.*, 50 to 60°, but is directed 30° caudally. This angle is adjusted until the tip of the needle is level with, and adjacent to, the posterior aspect of the L5-S1 disc space (Fig. 10.27). The relationship of the needle to the vertebral bodies is again of great importance in assessing bony obstruction. Obstruction by the transverse process necessitates complete repositioning of the needle. Obstruction by the pars interarticularis or facet joint necessitates reducing the angle of the needle closer to the sagittal plane. There are occasions when a broad transverse process of L5 obstructs the approach. If this

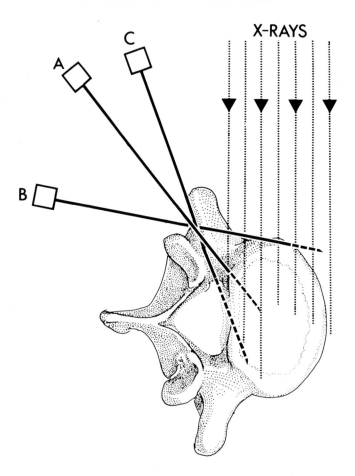

Figure 10.26. Diagrammatic representation of posterolateral approach to the disc space. *A*, correct approach; *B*, needle is off the edge of the disc space; and *C*, needle is entering foramen and possibly violating subarachnoid space.

problem is encountered, a more medial and inferior approach to needle insertion may be tried, placing the needle further posteriorly and inferior to the transverse process.

If there is unilateral sacralization of the transverse process of L5, the approach should be from the nonsacralized side. It is rare that you will be injecting chymopapain into such a disc.

Once the 4-inch No. 18 needle is positioned, a 6-inch No. 22 needle is passed through its lumen. The terminal ½ to ¾ inch of the No. 22 needle is bent, so that the bevel is on the convex aspect of the curve. It is advanced to the point that, when it emerges from the No. 18 needle, its bend will take it towards the L5-S1 disc space. If either bony margin of the disc space is encountered, the bevel is turned to face the bone. With

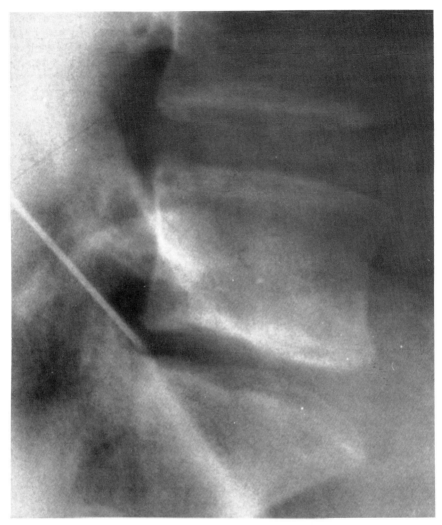

Figure 10.27. Four-inch, 18-gauge needle in position behind the L5-S1 disc space.

a narrowed L5-S1 disc space, localization of the tip of the needle and guidance into the disc space may only be achieved by alternating the image intensifier between the lateral and anteroposterior positions.

HIGHER LUMBAR DISC SPACES

The needle in the L4-5 disc space may be used as a guide to needle insertion above this level, and the technique employed is identical to that used for the L4-5 disc space. For the L3-4 disc space, a site 1 inch cephalad to the insertion site of L4-5 is selected. The L2-3 space is approached from approximately the same cephalocaudal level as that for the L3-4 space, but slightly closer to the midline. Usually, the 18-gauge, 6-inch needle can be inserted into these spaces, but occasionally the angle of insertion is such that a "piggyback" arrangement of needles, similar to that of the L5-S1 space, is required.

INSERTION OF SINGLE NEEDLE FOR SINGLE DISC SPACE INJECTION

To start your career in lateral lumbar discography and discolysis, you probably should put a needle in L4-5 (the easiest space to enter) as a marker. Using the L4-5 needle as a guide, entry into the L5-S1 disc space is facilitated. However, once you become adept at getting a needle into L5-S1, you should eliminate entry into other disc spaces when not clinically indicated.

USE OF THE BEVEL ON THE NEEDLE

It is best to aim for the middle of the disc on lateral x-ray. Occasionally you will be a shade too high and will encounter the lower edge of a vertebral body. Simply turning the bevel of the needle as in Figure 10.28 may allow you to compensate for this slight error.

A similar reverse exercise will sometimes get you into the disc space when you are too low in your approach.

In placing the needle in the "middle" of the disc, the bevel of the needle can be used as a chisel to direct the needle tip to the center of the disc.

CHANGING THE ANGLE OF NEEDLE INSERTION

The following are some final minor points on getting the needle into the disc space:
a. Needles do not turn corners when advanced over some distance. Look at Figure 10.29 and project a line from the end of the needle to the site of entry in the disc. The needle will not take the magical bend to enter the space; pull out and start again.
b. When changing direction of the needle, remember:
   i. You are changing the direction in two planes, but only one plane is showing on the screen.
   ii. A little change in direction means a lot of change in the ultimate position of the needle tip (Fig. 10.30).

CROSSING THE ANNULUS-NUCLEUS PLANES

We prefer dull needles for this procedure because of the tremendous feeling that comes from the nonsharp advancing needle tip. The feel of the annulus is much like that gritty feeling you had dancing on a floor covered with dance sand. The feeling from the nucleus is like cutting a piece of butter just removed from the refrigerator. The transition from dancing on sand to cutting hard butter is there to feel and always tells us we have positioned our needle tip in the nucleus pulposus.

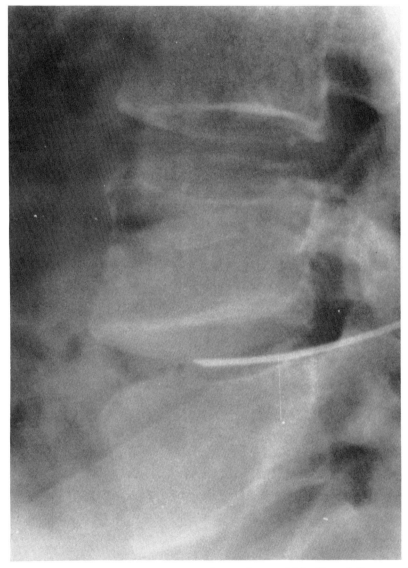

Figure 10.28. Bevel of 18-gauge needle used as a "chisel" to deflect needle into center of the disc space.

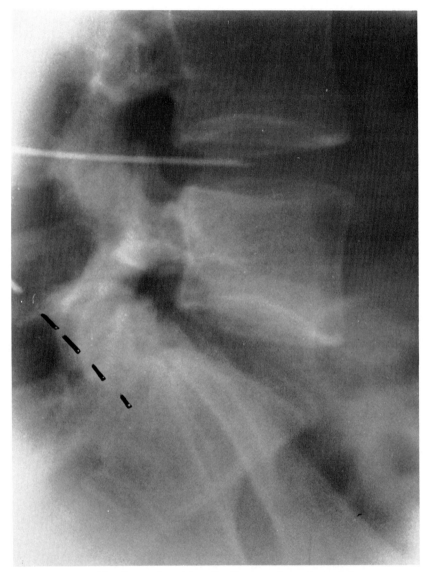

Figure 10.29. Needle approaching L5-S1, too low. *Dotted line* projection shows the position is too low. Remove the needle and begin again.

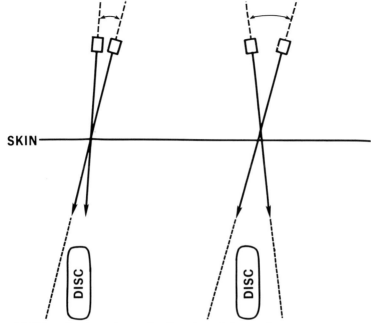

Figure 10.30.   A *minor* change in direction of the needle means a *major* change in the ultimate position of the needle tip.

Position of the Needle Tip in the Disc.

Figure 10.31 shows perfect positioning of needles in L4-5 and L5-S1. Note that the needle tip is in the center of the disc on lateral and anteroposterior and in the middle of the disc, halfway between each end plate. The acceptable standard for needle tip placement is the middle third of the disc on lateral, between the medial borders of the pedicles on anteroposterior (Fig. 10.32) and not under, or directed into, the end plate (Fig. 10.33). It is useful to take an x-ray with the image intensifier as a record of needle placement.

REPRODUCING LEG PAIN BEFORE YOU ARE IN THE DISC SPACE (STRIKING THE NERVE ROOT)

There are three ways you may reproduce leg pain before you are actually in the disc space and doing discometry. The most common way is to get your needle tip too high and too anterior to the disc space (Fig. 10.34), striking the nerve root. The second and most dangerous way is to advance towards the disc space in too vertical a direction and enter the foramen and dural sac (Fig. 10.35). The third and least disconcerting way is to have your needle perfectly positioned for entry into the symptomatic disc space, but each time you advance it you reproduce leg pain. We feel this represents mechanical stimulation of adhesions between the annulus and the nerve root (sciatica is usually on the same side as entry) and palpation of the annulus reproduces pain.

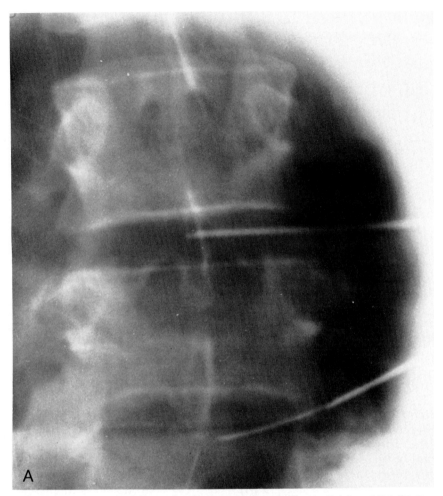

A

Figure 10.31. *A* and *B*, perfect positioning of needles in L4-5 and L5-S1 disc spaces. On anteroposterior view, the needle tip at L5-S1 appears buried in the end plate. This is because of the obliquity of the L5-S1 space on anteroposterior exposure.

In the first two cases, you must change the angle of advancement of the needle tip. In the last situation, gently advance the needle across the annulus into proper position. A little local anesthetic at this point may help.

RADIATION EXPOSURE

After reading this long technical discussion, you may feel that radiation exposure to the operating surgeon is extensive. Once the technique is learned, the radiation exposure for each case is between 10 and 15 seconds, much less than a radiologist receives in a barium enema or gastrointestinal series.

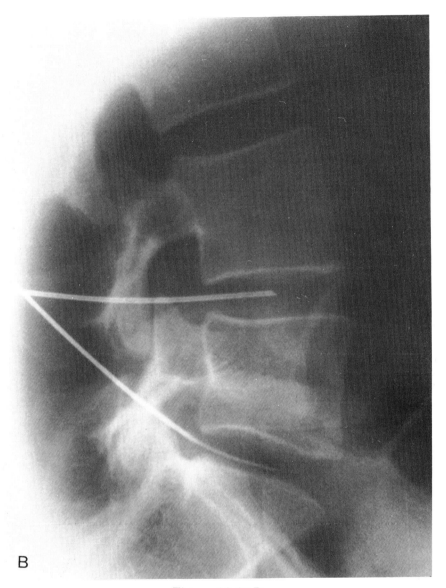

Figure 10.31*B*.

Discometry

Once the needles are in place such that the tip is in the mid-position on lateral radiography and between the medial borders of pedicles on anteroposterior (preferable midline), it is time to test the integrity of the disc space.

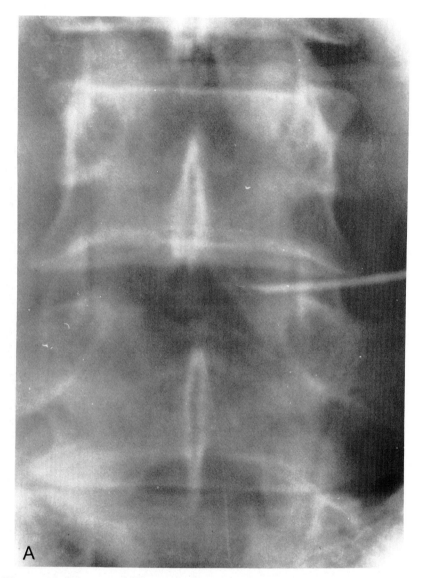

Figure 10.32. *A* and *B*, marginally acceptable needle position on anteroposterior and lateral views. Anteroposterior—needle tip just medial to pedicle; lateral—needle tip approaching the anterior one-third of the disc space.

There are three components to discography that require interpretation:
a. Pattern of contrast material.
b. Volume of test material that can be injected and resistance to injection.
c. Patient's response to the injection of the test material.

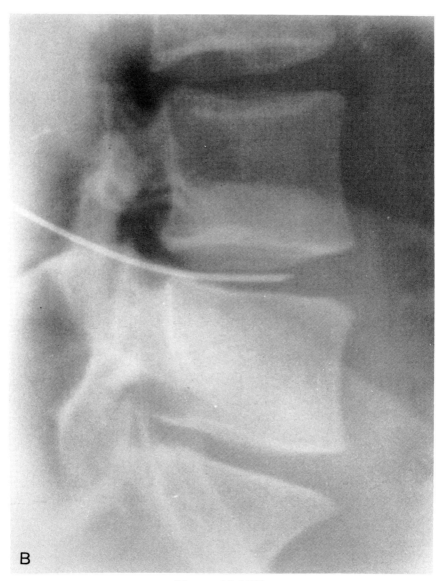

Figure 10.32*B*.

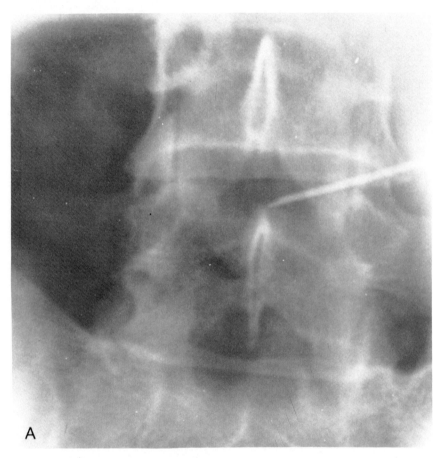

A

Figure 10.33. *A* and *B*, needle tip buried in the superior end plate of L5. This is an unacceptable position.

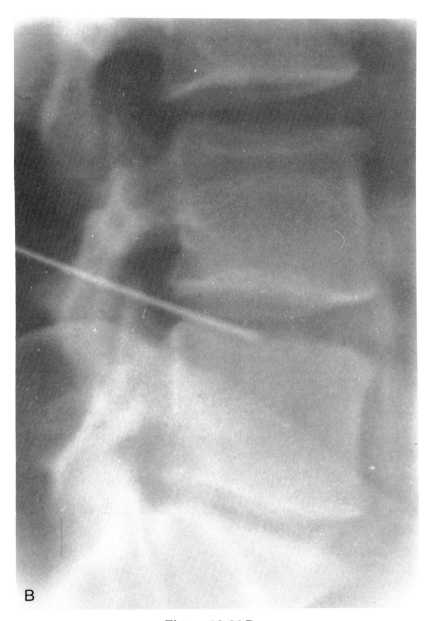

Figure 10.33*B*.

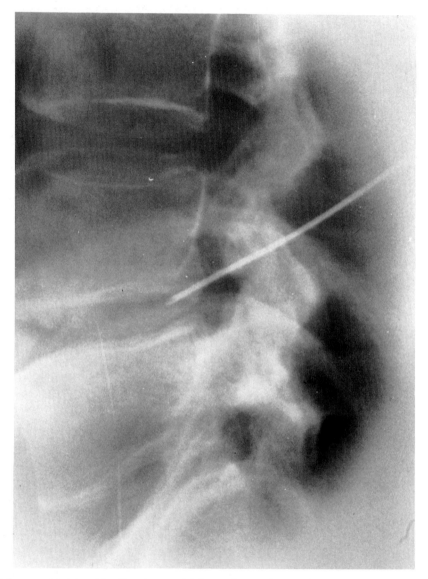

Figure 10.34. Needle tip too high, and anterior to line joining posterior vertebral borders, without the "feel" of the annulus. This is the most common cause of nerve root penetration.

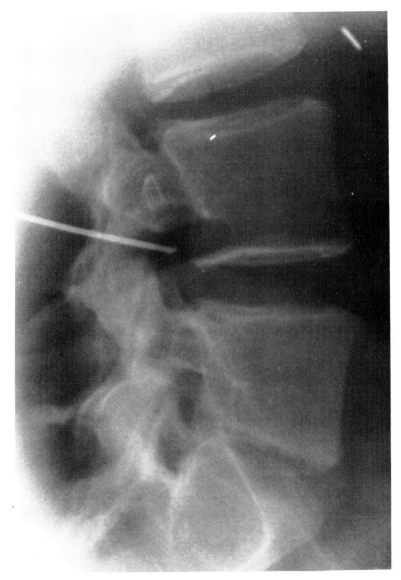

Figure 10.35.   Needle entering foramen. Further advancement would result in dural puncture and return of CSF. In this event, the procedure must be terminated.

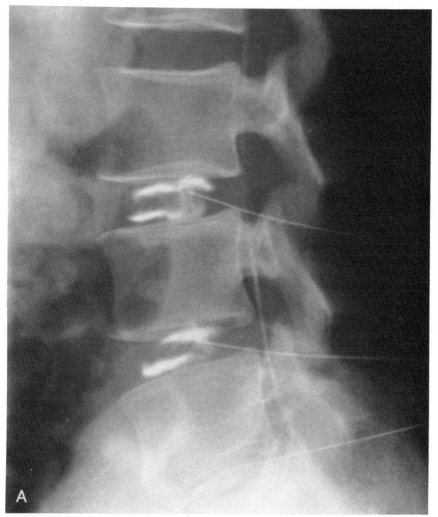

Figure 10.36. Normal disc patterns: *A*, "cookie sandwich"; *B*, cotton ball. The third normal pattern ("pancake") is represented in Figure 10.38 (L4-5).

PATTERN OF CONTRAST MATERIAL

There is no mistaking a normal disc; three patterns are seen (Fig. 10.36). The pattern and direction of leak of contrast material in a degenerative and/or herniated disc is shown in Figures 10.37 and 10.38.

The authors feel this is the least important of the three interpretive components. Our diagnosis of a herniated nucleus pulposus is firmly grounded in clinical criteria and supportive myelographic, venographic, or CT scanning procedures to the exclusion of discography. There are too many potential errors (6) in interpreting discographic patterns to

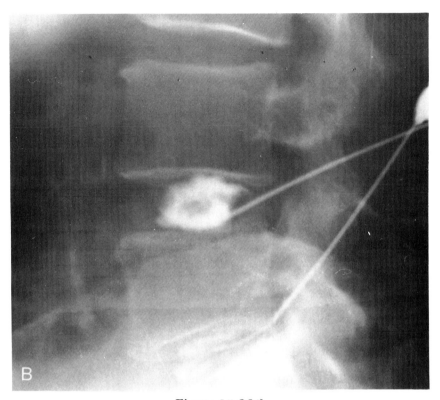

Figure 10.36B.

make it part of our criteria of selection of patient for chemonucleolysis. It is also felt that chymopapain should be injected into as "clean" a disc space as possible so that nothing, such as contrast material, is present to interfere with the action of chymopapain. There is no universal agreement on this point; in fact, Naylor and co-workers (7) have shown *in vitro* that there may be some enhancement of chymopapain activity by water-soluble contrast material. In spite of this evidence, it is our opinion that as little contrast material as possible be used (0.1 to 0.2 ml or preferably none) to identify the needle tip position. Identification of the site of the needle tip can sometimes be difficult at L5-S1, in a large patient using less than ideal imaging techniques. In this situation, it is mandatory that contrast material be used to identify the location of the needle tip.

With minimal or no use of contrast material, a radiographic pattern is not available for interpretation and discography *per se* is not completed.

VOLUME OF TEST MATERIAL THAT CAN BE INJECTED AND RESISTANCE TO INJECTION

The authors use the same material to test disc integrity as they use to constitute the chymopapain solution, *i.e.*, distilled water; thus, discography becomes discometry.

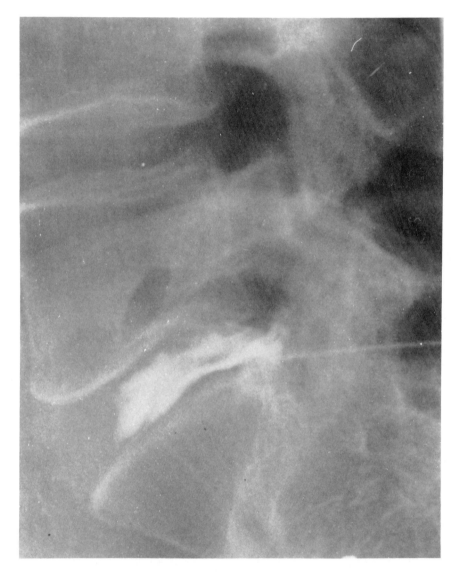

Figure 10.37.   Degenerative disc pattern at L5-S1.

A normal disc will rarely take up to 2 ml in volume. The younger the patient and the more "normal" the nucleus, the less can be injected, *i.e.*, in the 15- to 25-year-old age group, often 0.5 to 1.0 ml is all that will be accepted by the disc.

Every lumbar disc can accept some test material. On occasion a difficult needle placement will result in a plug of material (bone) blocking the end of the needle. On attempting to inject test material into the disc, firm resistance is met and *nothing* can be injected. This should not be

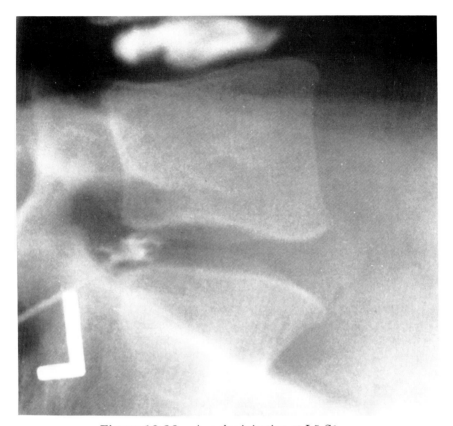

Figure 10.38. Annular injection at L5-S1.

interpreted as representing a normal disc. Rather the needle should be removed, unplugged with force, and reinserted.

A similar sensation of firm resistance is met with an injection into the annulus. However, some material can be injected and the typical pattern of annular injection is evident with the initial use of contrast material (Fig. 10.38).

The resistance met when injecting a normal disc is unquestionably firm. At times material will rebound out of the disc back into the syringe. If you are using a glass syringe to inject a normal disc you will break the glass syringe before you will break down the resistance of the disc.

The next level of resistance to injection (and thus restriction on volume that can be injected) is encountered in the disc that has been damaged through repetitive compressive loads or a single compressive load. The incomplete annular degeneration and tear occurs from the inside and nucleus migration is a protrusion only. This contained disc will accept more than normal amounts of test material and the clinically experienced symptoms will be reproduced. Theoretically, an annular tear that is complete can heal and the sealing of this "blowout" will increase resistance to injection and thus limit the amount of test material that can be injected. On rare occasions the incomplete or sealed annulus will "blow out" at the time of discometry and a small "popping" sensation will be noted.

The final level of resistance to discometry is almost no resistance at all. Large volumes of test material can be injected and escape through a complete tear in the annulus and into the extradural space. Only the conscious patient's pain response limits the volume to be used.

When confronted with a very large myelographic defect that may be indicative of a large disc herniation, it is prudent to limit the volume of test material injected to prevent any compromise of the cauda equina.

THE PATIENT'S RESPONSE TO INJECTION

The most important component to discometry is the patient's response to injection. Reproduction of pain in the extremity affected by sciatica is reassuring with regard to your diagnosis and needle position. Interestingly, failure to reproduce typical leg pain with discometry does not appear to lead to a poor result from chemonucleolysis.

When trying to reproduce leg pain, be satisfied with production of discomfort radiating into the buttock or leg on the symptomatic side. If only buttock discomfort occurs, without leg pain, stop testing the disc and accept the fact that you have lateralized discometry discomfort to the symptomatic side. Further, when assessing the patient's response to discometry, ask the patient about symptom reproduction in the following manner:

- "Am I producing pain or discomfort in the area of your buttock or leg where you normally feel your pain?"

Do not ask:

- "Am I producing the same pain as your sciatica?"

This latter question represents two questions to the patient: 1) Is the pain in the same location? and 2) Is it the same pain? It is sometimes necessary to inject large volumes of test material to produce a state that allows the patient to answer question 2. This is a state of extreme discomfort for a patient with acute sciatica and is unnecessary. It is this extreme state of pain that gives discography its poor reputation among patients.

It is suggested that, if it has been decided to perform two level discometry, the least symptomatic level clinically should be tested first. If you inject the most symptomatic level first, you may produce so much discomfort for the patient that any subsequent discometry is invalidated by the patient's continuing pain.

INTERPRETATION OF DISCOMETRY

Two factors are obvious. The supreme test of disc integrity is a discogram. Once you have demonstrated a normal disc through discography (Fig. 10.36) or discometry (a firm end point after 1.0 to 2.0 ml injection and no pain response from the patient), any myelographic "defect" or CT scan "shadow" can be set aside as a false positive.

Secondly, failure to reproduce *leg* pain at the time of discometry has no effect on the ultimate outcome from chemonucleolysis (8), providing your needle tip is correctly placed in the center of the disc.

Discometry is done for one purpose: to verify that your needle tip is in the correct nucleus and in the correct position. Reproduction of the patient's leg pain at the time of discometry is the supreme test of the needle's being in the right position in the correct nucleus. Failure to reproduce the patient's leg pain, and only to reproduce back pain, can easily be supported by the clinical setting of dominant leg pain, neurological symptoms, marked reduction in straight leg raising, neurological signs, and a positive myelogram or CT scan that led you to the decision to do chemonucleolysis on that particular disc.

Preparation and Injection of Chymopapain

Chemonucleolysis is accomplished by the injection of chymopapain (we have used Discase, Travenol Laboratories) at the time of discometry or discography. The material comes in a dried, lyophilized form and must be mixed to a 5-ml volume with distilled water according to the packaged instructions. Fifteen minutes after discography or a few minutes after discometry, 2 ml (8 mg or 5 nanokals) are injected into each disc. (If you wish to use contrast material, this 15-minute interval allows for the separation of contrast medium allergic reactions from chymopapain allergic reactions. The interval also allows for some dispersal of the contrast material and lessens its diluent effect on the chymopapain.)

It is advisable to inject chymopapain over the space of 2 to 3 minutes in order to allow for wide dispersal of the solution.

One syringe is used for each disc injection, because there are occasions when disc material is returned into the syringe at the time of chymopapain injection and this may serve to denature the chymopapain remaining in the syringe. Consequently, for multiple disc injections, it is important not to draw all the chymopapain solution from the vial into one syringe at once.

Chymopapain is bound instantly to the ground substance of nucleus pulposus. Thus, the needle can be removed soon after injection. The only caution is the occasion when, after injection, the chymopapain automatically refluxes into the syringe as a milky solution. If this occurs, the syringe should remain attached to the end of the needle and the refluxing chymopapain held in the disc space for 2 to 3 minutes. Pressure is then removed from the barrel of the syringe and any refluxed chymopapain is gathered in the syringe. The syringe is then removed, followed by the needle.

The authors do not feel that the water used for discometry has any adverse dilutional effect on the 2 ml of chymopapain injected.

POSTINJECTION IN THE OPERATING ROOM

Immediately after the injection, the conscious patient is rolled onto a stretcher in the supine position and observed for mild reactions. These include "tingling" and mild hypotension. The "tingling" sensation, or "prickling" as some patients describe it, starts in the face and spreads throughout the rest of the body. It follows circulation time and obviously represents a local reaction to the chymopapain or byproducts of disc dissolution, which quickly enter the bloodstream. On occasion, this sensation may be accompanied by a brief and minor episode of hypotension which requires no treatment. Both of these reactions are usually over within 2 to 3 minutes of the injection.

Anaphylactic reactions will almost always occur within 15 minutes of the injection of chymopapain. Many occur within a few minutes of the injection and are an extension of the minor reaction described above. However, the hypotension is unmistakably profound and is often associated with cold clammy skin, nausea, vomiting, skin rash, and other shock symptoms, such as light-headedness and shivering. Interestingly, all the patients remain conscious, and respiratory distress is usually nonexistent and, on occasion, will be described only as a "sensation of weight" on the chest. More will be said about anaphylaxis in Chapter 12, "Adverse Reactions to Chymopapain."

SUMMARY OF TECHNIQUE

1. Position, position, position.

   The three most common mistakes you will make in placing the needle correctly are:

   1. The patient will move out of position.
   2. The patient will move out of position.
   3. The patient will move . . . !

   This is the hardest lesson of all to learn.
2. Pick the correct disc:
   a. Know which root and which disc.
   b. See the front of sacrum.
   c. Watch congenital lumbosacral anomalies.
3. Select the proper entry site for injection of local anesthetic.
4. Place the needle properly—know your angles and bevels and center the needle tip in the nuclear space.
5. Appreciate the intricacies of discometry, discography.
6. Inject correct amount of active chymopapain into a clean disc space.

References

1. McCulloch JA, Ferguson JM: Outpatient chemonucleolysis. *Spine* 6:606, 1981.
2. Anderson N, Johansen SJ: Incidence of catecholamine induced arrhythmias during halothane anesthesia. *Anesthesiology* 24:51, 1963.
3. Lindblom K: Diagnostic puncture of intervertebral discs in sciatica. *Acta Orthop Scand* 17:231, 1948.
4. McCulloch JA, Waddell G: Lateral lumbar discography. *Br J Radiol* 51:498, 1978.

5. Froning N: Personal communication.
6. Holt EP: The question of lumbar discography. *J Bone Joint Surg* 50A:720, 1968.
7. Naylor A, Garland C, Robinson J: The effects of diagnostic radiopaque fluids used in discography on chymopapain activity. Presented at The International Society for The Study of The Lumbar Spine, Toronto, June 1982.
8. McCulloch JA: Chemonucleolysis. *J Bone Joint Surg* 59B:45, 1977.

CHAPTER 11

Post-Chemonucleolysis Course

The most important thing to know about the postinjection course is how variable it is. Some patients will have virtually no discomfort and others will have significant discomfort (usually backpain) that makes it impossible to leave the hospital for 1 or 2 days.

The postinjection course will be discussed on the assumption that the procedure was done under local, mild neuroleptic anesthesia without general anesthesia and intubation.

IMMEDIATE POSTINJECTION COURSE (0 TO 12 HOURS)
Back Pain

Our experience is to keep the patient in the recovery room for at least 60 minutes, observing for any untoward reactions. During that time most patients will notice some degree of back pain. The pain is nonmechanical in nature and persists regardless of the position of the patient. During the first hour in the recovery room, the patient usually receives an intramuscular injection of narcotic medication.

From this point the patients will follow one of three courses. The most common course is that as the first 12 hours go by the back pain increases slightly in severity but not beyond the point where standard amounts of analgesic medication fail to control symptoms. If patients have been preconditioned to expect this, they can cope with the pain. An uncommon course (perhaps 10% of the patients) is almost no discomfort at all. These patients will develop a minor low back pain that may not require any analgesia. Approximately 20% of the patients will follow a course of severe back pain, often described as spasms that virtually lock the patient into a position in bed. Any attempt to move is followed by severe, incapacitating back pain and muscle spasm over the entire back.

At this juncture it is important to emphasize three things:

1. As the pain increases after injection, the patients usually become apprehensive. They associate a minor procedure such as an injection with minor amounts of pain. The increasing discomfort in some, in spite of preconditioning, alarms them. They need constant reassurance in the first 1 or 2 days that the back pain they are witnessing postinjection is not unusual and will improve.
2. Most patients will notice improvement in their back discomfort if they get out of bed and walk. Within a few hours of the procedure, we suggest you ambulate most of the patients. There are a few who will have such significant discomfort in the back that they cannot walk immediately, but they should be encouraged to move as soon as possible.
3. Most patients require a light canvas corset to assist in ambulation.

In the majority of patients the back pain following chemonucleolysis is less than the back pain following laminectomy-discectomy. But be prepared for some patients to have tremendous back discomfort requiring complete bed rest, strong analgesia, and muscle relaxants. We have no theories as to why this reaction occurs except to suspect a postinjection reaction within the disc space that may include hemorrhage and may behave just as any other joint full of blood. We have considered the theory of dural irritation from chymopapain leaking through a rent in the annulus into the extradural space, but the pain is mechanical in nature and not increased by neck flexion.

Leg Pain

If the patient is going to get a good result from chemonucleolysis, the majority will notice an immediate "alteration" in their leg pain. Notice that we use the word alteration rather than relief because there are components of sciatica that will persist for days or weeks following injection. The sharpness and real discomfort of sciatica is what disappears immediately. The deep cramping sensation in the calf and sometimes in the buttock will persist for days or weeks. The paresthetic discomfort in the foot will persist for weeks.

Miscellaneous Immediate Postinjection Observations

If the patient is going to have an anaphylactic reaction, it will occur in the operating room or the recovery room. We have not had an anaphylactic reaction occur after 30 minutes. This will be discussed further in Chapter 12.

Some patients will experience nausea and vomiting. We have not been able to decide if this is a mild reaction to chymopapain or to the anesthetic or analgesic drugs used. It is so minor and readily treated that it has not been a problem. Occasionally a patient experiences lower abdominal cramps, thought to be due to irritation of the anterolongitudinal ligament. Again this has been a minor problem requiring no specific treatment.

INTERMEDIATE POSTINJECTION COURSE (12 HOURS TO 7 DAYS)
Back Pain

In this intermediate period, back pain becomes more tolerable to the patient. Usually by 2 to 3 days the requirement for analgesia starts to decrease and by the end of the first week the majority of patients do not require much more than 30 mg of codeine once or twice a day to control their discomfort. Again the variability in patient response and discomfort is emphasized.

The amount of back pain postinjection is the determining factor in postinjection ambulation, hospital discharge, and return to work. Most patients can be ambulated with brace support in the first 24 hours and most patients can be discharged from the hospital in 24 to 48 hours. Some patients have high levels of occupational demand, whether generated by the job situation or by the patient's motivation, and return to work within the first week. This is not recommended as a routine although the authors believe there is no harm in this quick return to activity. Most patients who follow this course will admit, in retrospect, that a return to work in this intermediate period was difficult and uncomfortable.

On occasion a patient may notice persistent sciatic scoliosis. We have had patients who have noticed a return of sciatic scoliosis immediately after chemonucleolysis. (These patients usually have had a sciatic scoliosis at some time in the past.) In both situations, the passage of time and the subsequent institution of exercises will lead to resolution of the scoliosis over a period of weeks.

Leg Pain

The course of leg pain following chemonucleolysis is so variable that it is impossible to draw conclusions about persisting leg pain in this intermediate period. It is most rewarding to see the smile on the patient's face who describes immediate relief of sciatica. But for those in whom leg symptoms persist, we suggest simple supportive observations for the first month. During that time, the following reactions may be noted:

1. The cramping sensation in the buttock and calf will gradually disappear.
2. The paresthetic discomfort in the foot will disappear.
3. "Rebound" leg pain may appear in the first few days. Previously, these patients were subjected to laminectomy because we thought this represented failure of enzymatic digestion of the nucleus. The common finding was mucoid-like material containing inflammatory cells which was thought to be residual, partially digested disc material. Recent experience shows that most of these patients improve, and it is not necessary to carry out an immediate laminectomy.
4. Pain in the opposite leg may occur infrequently. This is probably due to annular buckling causing tension on the opposite nerve root. Again, it is rarely the cause of failure unless a large central or midline sequestered disc is the cause of opposite leg pain.
5. The most unusual postinjection leg pain course is one of increasing severe leg pain over the first 1 to 4 days, becoming almost intolerable to the patient. This has occurred in less than 0.1% of patients over our decade of experience with the drug. Immediate surgical exploration has invariably revealed a large sequestrated disc. We have theorized that a long-standing extrusion which has become predominantly collagenous has been propelled into the spinal canal by the volume of material injected, thereby hydraulically producing sequestration of disc material, or worsening the extent of migration of a sequestered fragment.

Miscellaneous Intermediate Postinjection Observations

Most miscellaneous reactions will disappear during this intermediate phase. Nausea and vomiting, lower abdominal cramps, and back spasms always disappear during this interval.

During this time a delayed hypersensitivity reaction (hives) will appear in about 3% of patients (*cf.* Chapter 12).

LONG-TERM POSTINJECTION COURSE (1 MONTH PLUS)
Back Pain

Back pain has almost always subsided to a significant degree by the end of the first month following injection. At this stage most patients are prepared to shed their corset support and become more active. Except for patients engaged in heavy labor, most patients return to office duties and light household chores by this stage. Some exercise activity should be initiated at this juncture and all patients are instructed to gradually increase occupational and leisure activities. By 3 months, those patients who will obtain a good result will be very comfortable, up to most demands of life, and can be discharged from follow-up care. It is interesting to study these patients a few years later when many state that back discomfort continued to improve beyond the 3-month interval. During this stage, while muscular tone and control of the low back is being regained, the patient's final back symptom will be a sensation of weakness. In early stages some patients will describe sudden weakness or "giving way" in their back which is not associated with pain. As time passes this "giving way" sensation becomes simply weakness which in turn gives way to good back function.

Leg Pain

The patient who is going onto a good result will be free of leg pain at 1 month. Straight leg raising will be approaching normal. (We do not do straight leg raising testing in the first month because we feel it upsets the healing process occurring in the disc/root area.) Neurological recovery will occur in approximately 25% of these patients. For some it will be quick and dramatic; for most it will be slow and variable with little change noted at 1 month.

Some patients will be satisfied with the improved state of leg comfort but will still have vague sensations in their leg, usually in the form of calf cramping. These patients will have persistent reduction in straight leg raising although it will be improved over the preinjection state. These symptoms and signs gradually improve over the next few months.

In some patients vague leg sensations and straight leg raising reduction persist. Although they consider themselves improved, we feel they still have a mass of collagenous material beneath the nerve root or a lateral recess stenosis and will subsequently (months or years) have symptoms of recurrent sciatica.

HOW FAST DOES CHYMOPAPAIN WORK?

Chymopapain's effect on the nucleus is immediate, often seen by the reflux of milky hydrolyzed nuclear material that returns into the syringe at the time of injection. *In vivo* and *in vitro* experiments (Chapter 8, Refs. 1, 6, and 7) have shown that chymopapain is bound instantly to nuclear material and has an instant effect.

The real question is how fast are the effects of chemonucleolysis noticed by the patient? Many patients notice immediate relief of leg pain. It is likely that these patients have a significant proteoglycan, H_2O component to their herniated nucleus pulposus (HNP), and rapid hydrolysis deflates the HNP and quickly relieves sciatica. Other patients may not notice relief of sciatica for a number of weeks. These patients may have a greater collagen component to their disc herniation. We do not feel that chymopapain works by damaging nerves (such as sinuvertebral) because the dramatic relief in pain occurs in the leg, not the back. Further, experimental work (1) has shown that bathing rabbit nerves in chymopapain has no effect on nerve structure or function.

The scarring or fibrosis across the disc space takes many months to mature to the point where back pain disappears as a symptom.

How fast does chymopapain work? Immediately. How soon will the patient notice the effect? Days to weeks for leg pain; weeks to months for back pain.

RADIOGRAPHIC ASSESSMENT

It has been our routine to x-ray patients 1 month after chemonucleolysis. Any disc space narrowing that is to appear will be apparent at this stage. This disc space narrowing occurs gradually over the first month and rarely increases after that. It is difficult to accept that such profound disc space narrowing can occur without such sequelae as lateral recess stensois or facet joint syndromes but our experience has been just that.

On occasion a discitis reaction is seen on x-ray (Fig. 11.1). These patients usually have prolongation of back pain but eventually and most often it becomes asymptomatic. Disc space infection following chemonucleolysis has occurred very infrequently as a clinical syndrome, and in our series we have not had a patient with a proven disc space infection (fever and a positive culture from the disc or the bloodstream). Perhaps any bacteria that would venture into the disc space at the time of injection of chymopapain would immediately have its cell wall dissolved.

FAILURE

If, at 1 month following injection, the patient still has the same or disabling *leg* pain, the procedure is considered a failure and surgery is recommended. *Back* pain at this stage may still be a complaint, but the patient should be encouraged to live with it for a further few months before considering the chemonucleolysis a failure.

If you are selecting the correct patient for chemonucleolysis, the most common reason for failure will be a sequestered disc. It follows that if the patient has a sequestered disc one of two situations prevail. The disc is truly sequestered and chymopapain injected into the disc space cannot reach the fragment or, secondly, chymopapain, on injection, leaks into the extradural space only to encounter a predominantly collagenous mass of sequestrated disc, upon which it has no effect.

The second most common cause of failure is lateral recess stenosis which probably predated the injection of chymopapain. The patient may

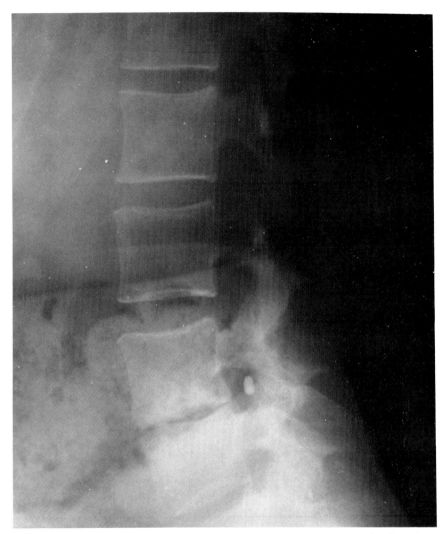

Figure 11.1. Discitis 6 months post-chemonucleolysis. At 3 months there were early changes. At 6 months the patient has minimal nocturnal discomfort, normal temperature and WBC, but a slightly elevated ESR, and a positive bone scan.

be seen as having an acute disc herniation with the sudden onset of dominant leg pain, neurological symptoms and signs, and significant straight leg raising reduction on the basis of a small disc protrusion compromising an already narrowed lateral recess. Chemonucleolysis decompression of this disc protrusion does not relieve the symptoms because of associated changes in the lateral recess or further narrowing of the lateral recess leading to continuing compromise of root function.

THE LATERAL RECESS FOLLOWING
CHEMONUCLEOLYSIS

Many find it hard to accept the fact that the severe disc space narrowing (Fig. 11.2) that occurs following chemonucleolysis does not cause pedicular kinking or some other form of lateral recess stenosis and

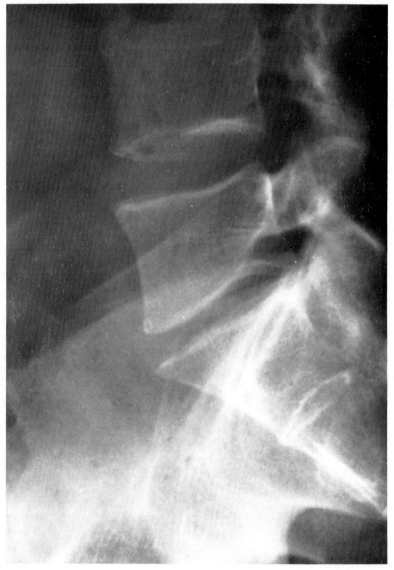

Figure 11.2. Disc space narrowing at L5-S1, 1 month following chemonucleolysis.

thus sciatica. Our experience has been that pedicular kinking and other forms of lateral recess stenosis causing symptoms do not occur long term. On long-term follow-up (2), we noticed an extremely low incidence of early or late recurrence of sciatica suggesting that lateral recess stenosis is not a complication.

Explanation for this is twofold. First, with descent of the vertebral body cephalad to the narrowed disc space occurs descent of every other vertebral body cephalad and the contents of the spinal canal. Thus, the pedicle does not get the opportunity to guillotine the nerve root. Secondly, narrowing of the disc space is associated with scarring of the disc. This builds in inherent stability, reducing movement at that segmental level and thus reducing the chance that any encroachment on root territory will become symptomatic through mechanical stimulation of movement (3).

In summary, the symptom of sciatica in lateral recess stenosis is due to encroachment and the mechanical stimulation through movement. Sciatica, due to lateral recess stenosis, does not occur short or long term because the compromise of root territory is minimal and is more than compensated for by the stability introduced to that segment by disc space narrowing and disc space fibrosis.

SURGERY FOLLOWING CHEMONUCLEOLYSIS

Surgery following chemonucleolysis has not been compromised or complicated by prior injection of chymopapain. The authors have operated on approximately 200 patients in whom chemonucleolysis failed and surgical intervention has been no different technically than the first open surgical procedure on any lumbar spine. There is no increased incidence of adhesions as has been stated by some.

If you are selecting your patients well for chemonucleolysis (which implies that most of your injections are single space injections), then the most common cause of chemonucleolysis failure will be the sequestered disc (approximately 50% of the failures). If the chymopapain injection in these cases has dissolved the intradiscal nuclear material and has narrowed the disc space as measured on a postinjection lateral radiograph, then the surgical management of a sequestered disc is very straightforward. Simply carry out a small laminectomy approach (microdiscectomy is recommended) and remove the sequestered fragment. Do not enter the disc space; it is unnecessary and upsets the interdiscal scar that is forming and stabilizing that segment.

The second most common cause of failure is usually lateral recess stenosis leaving the patient with persistent leg and back pain. The obvious question is whether this stenosis predated the chemonucleolysis and was misdiagnosed, or is it the result of chemonucleolysis and the disc space narrowing that occurs? The authors feel that the former is true, that lateral recess stenosis was present prior to the chemonucleolysis, perhaps with some further decompensation of the lateral recess by an annular bulge. Again, the surgical exercise is an extradiscal decompres-

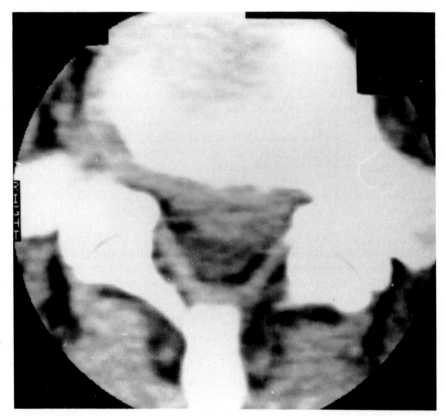

Figure 11.3.   CT scan showing a large HNP, L5-S1, left.

sion of the nerve root, leaving the maturing scar within the disc undisturbed.

The final cause of failure is persistent back pain with or without varying degrees of sciatica. The operative findings are usually nonspecific in this group of patients with varying degrees of small disc protrusions and minor root adhesions, no different than the adhesions seen in some patients who have first time surgery without prior injection of chymopapain into the lumbar spine. Surgical intervention in this group of patients involves more than root decompression and is not a topic for this monograph.

There is a rare occasion (0.1%) when chemonucleolysis is followed by a dramatic increase in leg pain which, from the day of injection, is almost intolerable to the patient. These patients require immediate discectomy at which time a large sequestered disc or fragment of end plate—annulus—will be found. As stated, we suspect that the hydraulic action of discometry has further pushed the extruded or sequestered disc fragment further into nerve root territory to cause the dramatic increase in sciatica. It is interesting to note the absence of further neurological compromise when this happens. (We have seen one exception to this—a patient who was worse neurologically.) Relief of sciatica following surgery in this infrequent situation has been quite dramatic.

The increase in back pain following chemonucleolysis is not to be seen as an indication of failure and thus a reason for surgical intervention. We stress that almost all patients should be followed for at least 1 month before the procedure can be considered a failure and surgical intervention occurs.

POST-CHEMONUCLEOLYSIS CT SCAN

The two most common investigative tools used prior to chemonucleolysis are myelography and CT scanning. Falconer and co-workers (4) pointed out many years ago the phenomenon of a persistent myelographic defect after sciatica is resolved.

Early in our experience with chemonucleolysis, we were also aware of a persistent myelographic defect following chymopapain injection and relief of symptoms. We had the occasion to leave oil contrast material in

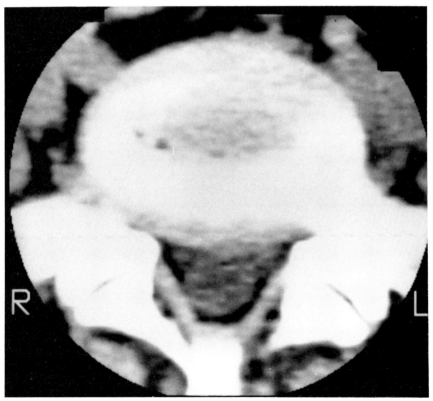

Figure 11.4.   Postinjection CT scan, showing the defect largely resolved.

the subarchnoid space of one patient and screened him on a regular basis (5). Symptoms were immediately relieved by the injection of chymopapain yet the myelographic defect persisted unaltered for 6 weeks. After 6 weeks it started to change and ultimately disappeared.

The most exciting information about investigative defects following chemonucleolysis is coming from CT scanning before and after chymopapain injection. Figure 11.3 shows a large HNP defect before chemonucleolysis. The patient noticed immediate relief of sciatica and 2 months later the CT scan shows that the defect has disappeared (Fig. 11.4).

Figures 11.5 & 6 show two patients, each with an HNP at L4–5. Each had outpatient chemonucleolysis after CT scan supported the diagnosis of an HNP causing sciatica. Both had immediate relief of sciatica and were back to their professional lives, full time, within 2 weeks of the

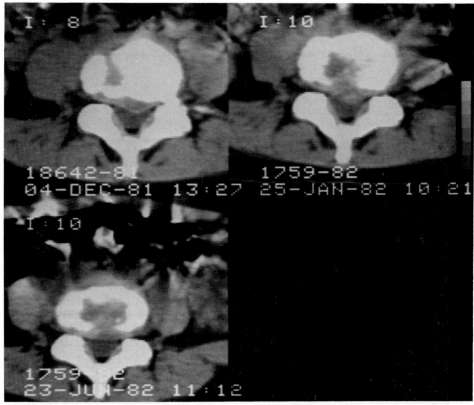

Figure 11.5.   Three CT scans: December 1981—preinjection, showing an HNP at L4-5; January 1982—1 month postinjection; June 1982—6-months postinjection. These demonstrate a persistent defect 1 month postinjection with relief of symptoms, and, without further treatment, the disappearance of the defect 5 months later.

injection. Post-chemonucleolysis CT scans in the first patient (Fig. 11.5) showed a persisting defect 1 month postinjection. CT scans 6 months, following chemonucleolysis showed further resolution of the defect. In the second patient CT scans within 2 months of the injection showed disappearance of the mass.

This observation supports the concept that the pain of sciatica is related to three factors: a) the mass of nuclear material that has herniated; b) the proteoglycan, H_2O distention within that mass of nuclear material; and c) an inflammatory reaction.

Chymopapain causes rapid hydrolysis of the proteoglycan complex and converts the distended "golf" ball to a "cotton" ball of collagen fibers. This residual collagenous "cotton ball" portion of the HNP is the reason for a persisting defect on CT scan. Ultimately, over a period of time and through the natural defense mechanisms of the body, the mass disappears. The inflammatory reaction is immediately altered by disc hydrolysis, just as it is altered with almost any fluid massage of the disc fragment or epidural space by saline or steroid (6, 7).

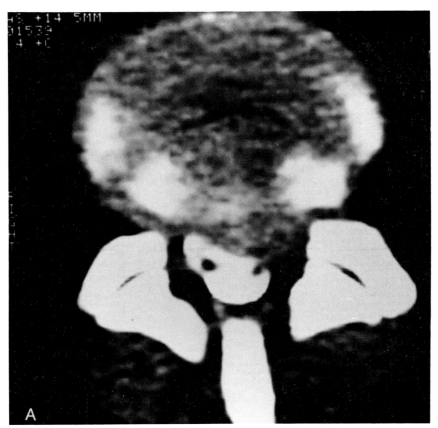

Figure 11.6.   *A*, augmented CT scan showing an HNP, L4-5, preinjection.

LONG-TERM RECURRENCE OF SYMPTOMS FOLLOWING SUCCESSFUL CHEMONUCLEOLYSIS

The recurrence rate, long term, after an initially successful chemonucleolysis is low (1.4%) (2).

The reasons for *recurrence of sciatica* are as follows:

1. The HNP is at the same level (same or opposite side). There are two possible explanations for this:
    a. The mass of HNP has not been completely resolved and with the passage of time, and possibly an injury, there is reestablishment of the inflammatory interface between the nerve root and the retained fragment, leading to recurrent symptoms.
    b. The disc reconstitutes itself and reherniates. We favor the former explanation.
2. The HNP is at a different level. The explanation for this is obvious.
    A patient cannot have a second injection and both these situations require operative intervention.
3. The recurrence of symptoms in the back or leg is related to some of the many other diagnoses listed in Table 7.1.

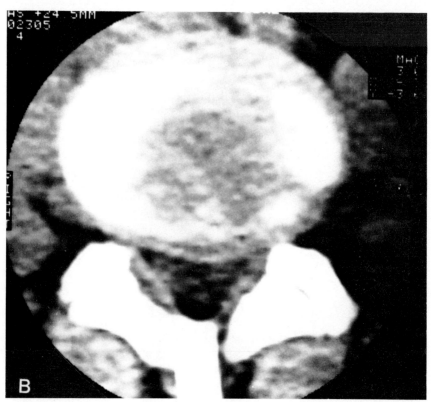

Figure 11.6.   *B*, postinjection CT scan.

SUMMARY

The most predictable thing about the post-chemonucleolysis course is its unpredictability. The most dramatic feature of the postinjection course is the immediate relief of sciatica. When this does not occur, patients become discouraged. Initially, we too, were discouraged but quickly learned not to intervene before 1 month postinjection.

Back pain will persist longer and must not be construed as an indication of failure for at least 3 months.

A long postoperative guide is included as an appendix to this monograph. Patients appreciate this outline which, in essence, tells them to use common sense during their first 3 months postinjection.

References

1. Hudson A, McKinnon S: Effect of chymopapain on peripheral nerve tissue. Personal communication on work to be published.
2. McCulloch JA: Chemonucleolysis for relief of sciatica due to a herniated intervertebral disc. *Can Med Assoc J* 124:880, 1981.
3. Bertolini J, Miller J, Spencer O: The effect of intervertebral disc space narrowing on the contact force between the nerve root and a simulated disc protrusion. Presented at the International Society for the Study of the Lumbar Spine, Toronto, June 1982.
4. Falconer MA, McGeorge M, Begg CA: Observations on the cause and mechanism of symptom production in sciatica and low back pain. *J Neurol Neurosurg and Psychiatry* 11:13, 1948.
5. Macnab I, *et al.*: Chemonucleolysis. *Can J Surg* 14:280, 1971.
6. Fraser R: Chymopapain for the treatment of intervertebral disc prolapse—A double blind study. Presented at the International Society for the Study of the Lumbar Spine, Toronto, June 1982.
7. Bernine P, Wiesel S, Feffer H, *et al.*: Effectiveness of epidural steroids in the treatment of sciatica—A double blind clinical trial. Presented at the International Society for the Study of the Lumbar Spine, Toronto, June, 1982.

CHAPTER 12

Adverse Reactions to Chymopapain

Chemonucleolysis is a safe procedure. Like any other procedure, troubles will quickly arise if you do not handle the drug and the procedure properly.

There are three situations where you will be guaranteed problems:

1. *Never cross the subarachnoid space with the needle that will be used to inject chymopapain.*

   The reason for this is simple: Chymopapain must never enter the subarachnoid space. It dissolves the basement membranes of the small vessels of the pia-arachnoid and the subarachnoid hemorrhage that follows may result in death, immediate unconsciousness, convulsions, or delayed fibrosis of the cauda equina (interfering with such vital functions as bowel and bladder control and lower extremity function).

   For the same reason you should separate any puncture of the subarachnoid space (*e.g.*, myelogram) and the injection of chymopapain that may leak into the extradural space. It is not uncommon that anything injected into the disc space through the lateral approach will leak out through a rent in the annulus into the extradural space. If a communication exists between the extradural space and the subarachnoid space, it is possible for chymopapain to pass through this communication into the subarachnoid space and cause problems. This communication can occur at the time of lateral discography when you are too vertical in your approach to the disc space and inadvertently enter the subarachnoid space. The flow of cerebrospinal fluid will tell you that you have committed this technical error. It should also tell you to stop the procedure and wait 48 hours for the dural puncture to seal before proceeding with chymopapain injection. Similarly, a dural puncture with a large bore needle for oil-soluble myelography or multiple dural punctures during a difficult myelogram should be followed by a similar 48-hour interval to allow for sealing of the communication between the extradural and subarachnoid spaces.

   Chymopapain must be injected through a needle that has been inserted into the disc through the posterolateral approach; do not use a midline approach.

2. *Do not inject chymopapain until you are sure the needle tip is in the nuclear area of a disc.*

   Chymopapain will not be of any value and indeed may be potentially harmful if injected directly into the tissues or structures outside the annulus fibrosis, such as the retroperitoneal space, bowel, large vessels or extradural space. You must know exactly where your needle tip is before injection; this may require the injection of contrast material and obtaining two views of the disc space at 90° to each other (see Chapter 10, Technique of Chemonucleolysis). Only when you are satisfied with the position of the tip of the needle should you inject chymopapain.

3. *Contraindications to chymopapain injection are clearly set out in the product brochure. Obey those instructions.*

   A. Patients who have had a prior injection of chymopapain may be sensitized to the drug and should not receive a repeat injection of chymopapain for fear of precipitating a significant anaphylactic reaction. Likewise, patients who have known sensitivity to chymopapain (food allergies) may have an increased risk of an allergic reaction and should not be injected.

   B. Patients with neurological disorders, especially those involving the spinal cord or peripheral nerves (*e.g.*, multiple sclerosis or acute paralysis of any origin) should not be subjected to possible adverse effects of chymopapain entering the spinal canal subsequent to injection into the disc space. Do not inject these patients.

   C. Pregnant women cannot be injected with chymopapain because no one knows the potential danger of chymopapain or disc dissolution products crossing the placenta.

   D. It has been stated that chymopapain should not be used in teenagers. We feel chymopapain can be used in 13- and 14-year-old patients with a documented herniated intervertebral disc. Fortunately, this is a rare clinical situation we have faced with excellent results and no adverse effects (1).

   E. Patients with significant cauda equina compression from a large central disc herniation or severe spondylolisthesis do not need any further volume compromise of their spinal canal. Do not inject chymopapain for fear that the volume injected may further compromise impaired neurological function.

   F. Do not perform chemonucleolysis at cord levels (above *L2*).

GENERAL CONTRAINDICATIONS

It may be stated that specific, unusual contraindications will occur. An example would be a patient with a recent myocardial infarct. Obviously, you would not inject chymopapain in this situation because of the possibility of anaphylaxis and hypotension causing the patient's demise. Other general medical contraindications may occur.

ADVERSE REACTIONS

Adverse reactions to, or following, chymopapain injection can be classified into two broad categories: sensitivity reactions and procedural related reactions (including neurological reactions).

Approximately 3% of patients who undergo chemonucleolysis will experience a complication. Providing you stay out of the subarachnoid space, all of these complications are treatable, self-limiting, and of no long-term consequence to the patient. The most serious complication is anaphylactic shock which occurs in 0.5% or less of patients (2). If you are prepared, with the patient in the operating room, an attending anesthesiologist, and a large bore cannula IV in place, you will meet the challenge.

Sensitivity Reactions

These are subclassified as:

Anaphylaxis
Angioneurotic edema
Rash (itching)
Urticaria
} These four hypersensitivity reactions can occur alone or in combination.

ANAPHYLAXIS

The most serious concern to the use of chymopapain is anaphylaxis. It is *the* complication that strikes the most fear in user's hands. To date, four deaths (3, 4) in other centers have occurred following chymopapain injection and an anaphylactic reaction. The junior author has had 15 anaphylactic reactions, representing an incidence of 0.35%. The authors have had no deaths.

We cannot emphasize enough:
1. At all times be prepared for anaphylaxis.
2. At all times be prepared for a profound reaction.
3. At all times be prepared to ask for immediate help from your anesthesiology and medical colleagues.

Anaphylaxisis is rapid in onset, profound in extent, and allows only minutes for the right decisions to be made.

Basic Science Considerations

Anaphylaxis is an immune response, occurring in a previously sensitized individual immediately following the injection of the appropriate antigen (plant protein chymopapain). The onset of the reaction is within minutes of injection. We have not witnessed an anaphylactic reaction beyond 30 minutes from the time of injection of chymopapain, with almost all of our reactions occurring immediately after injection while the patient is in the operating room.

Symptoms

Symptoms and signs of anaphylaxis in man are predominantly those of vascular shock. This occurs when the antigen-antibody reaction occurs on the previously sensitized mast cell resulting in the release of histamine and other vasoactive compounds. The major antibody involved is IgE which is bound to mast cells and circulating basophils. The major effect of histamine release in humans occurs on blood vessels resulting in an increase in vascular permeability and a shift of circulating volume from the intravascular to the interstitial space. It is likely that the H_1-receptors mediate most of these effects. The H_2-receptor-mediated effects on gastric secretion and heart rate are not as dramatic as the vasodilation and profound cardiovascular collapse. We have also been impressed with the lack of bronchiolar constriction and respiratory distress. Certainly angioneurotic edema and mild upper airway obstruction have been factors in one of our reactions, but in patients recently followed (2), not one required intubation.

Clinical Considerations

The management of the profound cardiovascular collapse is best carried out without the masking effects of drugs used in general anesthesia. Chemonucleolysis should be done under local anesthesia.

1. The reaction is profound and requires vigorous, rapid resuscitation. We prefer that the attending anesthesiologist administer the required medications and a second anesthesiologist oxygenate the patient by mask and monitor the vital signs. We feel this setting is best accomplished in an operating room rather than an x-ray facility. In the case of a reaction occurring in the recovery room we quickly move the patient back to the operating room for management.

   Chemonucleolysis should be performed in an operating room where adequate help is available for treating the emergency of anaphylaxis.

2. Often there is an early warning of a pending anaphylaxis. The conscious patient will report a sensation of tingling which follows circulation patterns, *i.e.*, neck, face, body, arms, and legs, in that order. Patients may report that they are suddenly nauseated or that their extremities are cold. This early warning system in the conscious patient often gives the anesthesiologist 1 to 3 minutes to prepare medication for treatment of anaphylaxis. Often the reaction will abort and anaphylaxis will not occur. It is rare that an anaphylactic reaction will occur without this warning.

   It is strongly suggested that chemonucleolysis should be performed with the patient conscious, so that the early warning symptoms can prompt early specific treatment.

3. The incidence of anaphylaxis is approximately 0.5%. This is a small number and for this reason routine premedication is not advised. Our concerns about premedication are sevenfold.

   a. An incidence of 0.5% means that 199 patients will receive unnecessary (albeit nonharmful) medication.

   b. There is no reported chemonucleolysis series where premedication has reduced the anaphylaxis rate below our incidence.

   c. Patients who have been premedicated according to suggested protocol (H_1 and H_2 blockers and steroids) have gone through severe anaphylactic reactions (5).

   d. Laboratory work in progress, in our center, with dogs sensitive to chymopapain suggests that premedication does not block, but may attenuate, the anaphylactic reaction.

   e. The most effective drug in the treatment of anaphylaxis is epinephrine. The risks of using this drug prophylactically far outweigh any potential benefits.

   f. Severe anaphylaxis requires aggressive treatment with large doses of medication. Premedication is low dose in nature and may alter or delay anaphylaxis, confusing the reaction and treatment.

g. The best defense for anaphylaxis is an alert, aggressive surgical-anesthetic team that has not been lulled into a false sense of security by premedication.

4. To date there is no pattern to the allergy history that will forewarn you that anaphylaxis is a threat (2). Patients with a long history of allergies have gone through the procedures with no untoward reactions and patients with no allergic history of any sort have had an anaphylactic reaction. Aside from the obvious history of an allergy to chymopapain or meat tenderizer, there appears to be no prior warning system. To date there is no proven screening test to detect reactors to chymopapain injection. *Every patient who undergoes chymopapain injection is at risk. Be prepared in every case to manage anaphylaxis.*

5. The classic anaphylactic reaction will be a profound and rapid drop in blood pressure (usually to 0 systolic), a diffuse body rash, cold, clammy skin, and nausea and vomiting in a conscious patient. Variations such as a partial drop in blood pressure with no body rash and no nausea or vomiting can occur. Additional reactions such as angioneurotic edema can occur and, in fact, the only time we have come close to respiratory distress was in a female patient with a profound anaphylactic reaction and the quick onset of angioneurotic edema including laryngeal edema. With quick intervention, her respiratory distress disappeared without anything other than oxygen by mask and an oropharyngeal airway being required.

Be prepared for any combination of clinical signs indicating anaphylaxis.

6. With one anesthesiologist managing the airway and monitoring the patient and another anesthesiologist administering to the patient, there are four cornerstones to management:

A. Epinephrine. Epinephrine is the first line of defense. It acts as an antagonist to histamine in various ways. It decreases the release of histamine from mast cells and inhibits the effect of histamine on vascular permeability and in turn prevents and reverses vascular collapse by increasing cardiac output.

Epinephrine (1/1000 solution) diluted to 10 ml is used intravenously. There is a difference of opinion whether epinephrine is used IM or IV, but the profound reaction has led us to intravenous use so that its effect is immediate. We measure its effect with blood pressure monitoring and cardiac monitoring, the latter to be sure we are not inducing cardiac arrhythmias.

There is also a difference of opinion as to what dose is to be used. We again stress the profound reaction and the necessity for adequate doses. It is generally recommended that for profound hypotension 2 ml of 1/10,000 solution be used. We have found that this is the minimum dose and in the usual significant reaction we are using doses of up to 5 ml in the first few minutes followed by further doses depending on the patient's response.

Warning: Do not overdose with epinephrine. The patient who is not hypotensive is very sensitive to epinephrine and hypertensive or cardiac arrhythmia complications can occur.

Do not underdose with epinephrine. The patient who is profoundly hypotensive (osystolic) is very resistant to epinephrine, *i.e.*, titrate the epinephrine dose very closely with blood pressure monitoring.

B. Antihistamines. Antihistamines inhibit the effects of histamines on the peripheral vascular tree. The effect is slower than that of adrenaline, but it is important to administer them immediately. We recommend an initial dose of 50 mg of Benadryl and we are prepared to administer 2 or 3 times that dose depending on the patient's response.

C. Cortisone. The rationale for the use of cortisone is less clear than for adrenaline and antihistamines. It is thought that cortisone will stabilize the mast cell membrane and inhibit the release of histamine. Its action is also slow. Our experience is that large doses are needed and we are quick to use 1 g of Solu-Cortef or equivalent.

D. IV Fluids. The shift of volume from the vascular to the extravascular space is profound. Be prepared to give large volumes of IV fluids in the form of crystalloid and colloid solutions. All the drugs in the world will not save a patient's life if you fail to realize how depleted in volume the intravascular space can become.

We routinely start a second IV infusion with a large bore catheter. We have recently had an occasion to start a third IV infusion in a patient in profound hypotension. We routinely *pump* in the crystalloid solution (usually Ringers-lactate for the first 4 liters). Our experience is that at least 4 liters of fluid is required in order to replenish the volume of the vascular space. We usually have this "on board" in approximately 15 minutes.

If you are dealing with an older patient, or a patient with an impairment of circulating volume dynamics (heart or kidney disease) you must insert a central venous pressure (CVP) line to monitor your attempts at replacing fluid volume. If you do not have the anaphylactic reaction resolved in a healthy young patient within 15 minutes after 4 liters of fluid replacement you must also insert a CVP line so that both arterial and venous pressures can be monitored. By this time your medical colleagues should be assisting you with advice regarding acid-base balance, the use of colloids (albumin), other crystalloids, and the necessity for other drugs such as bronchodilators.

It is our experience that most reactions, vigorously treated with adrenaline, antihistamines, cortisone, and large volumes of IV fluid are aborted in 15 minutes. But do not let your guard down after the initial resuscitation. We have seen patients go through repeated episodes of hypotension after initial successful resuscitation and require further vigorous treatment.

The junior author has treated 15 reactions so far with no serious long-term complications and no deaths (2). No patients required intubation. Twelve of the 15 patients went on to a good result to the injection of chymopapain.

Preinjection Testing

It seems only natural to prescreen patients undergoing chymopapain injection in an attempt to identify those patients who might react.

Skin Test. Recently we have been screening patients with a chymopapain skin test (6). Our test solution has been chymopapain solution left at room temperature (for 24 hours) to autodigest itself. It thus loses its enzymatic activity but maintains its antigenic activity. After mixing this solution in buffer (carbonate in 0.4% phenol) and suspending it in glycerol the standard skin test has been carried out in 300 consecutive patients. We have had a high percentage of patients with positive skin tests go on to some immediate allergic reaction (anaphylaxis, angioneurotic edema, skin reactions). Two patients with negative skin tests have experienced postinjection allergic reactions. We are continuing the skin test routine but are of the opinion that there is a reasonable, but not a perfect, degree of accuracy in using a skin sensitivity test to identify potential reactors to chymopapain.

Serological Test. We are actively monitoring patients pre- and postinjection with seriological testing for IgE and IgG antibodies to see if we can detect potential reactors. To date this work has not progressed to the point where we have clinically useful information (6).

ANGIONEUROTIC EDEMA

Most often this allergic reaction occurs in conjunction with anaphylaxis. It can occur by itself and there is then usually a minor delay of 15 minutes or a few hours as it builds in appearance. In our experience it has almost always started in the first 30 minutes after injection. It requires vigorous treatment with IV cortisone and antihistamines in doses similar to those used in the treatment of anaphylaxis. If there is any indication of an associated hypotension, the addition of IV fluids and epinephrine is mandatory.

Skin Rash and Itching

Alone or part of an anaphylactic reaction, the patient may develop a red lobster-like rash over the body. It is usually associated with itchiness and is readily handled by intravenous Benadryl. If it does not show signs of resolution within 15 minutes of administration of antihistamines (as measured by its appearance and the patient's sensation of itchiness), IV Solu-Cortef is added to the treatment routine. Any patient who goes through any of these immediate hypersensitivity reactions should be discharged home on a 1-week course of oral antihistamines.

Seven to 10 days postinjection, the patient may notice the sudden onset of urticaria or hives with itching. This is a minor reaction readily controlled with antihistamines. It is the most common reaction following chemonucleolysis, occurring twice as commonly as anaphylaxis.

Procedural Related Reactions

These are subclassified as: specific, including muscle spasm, discitis, and neurological damage (root or cauda equina with subsequent arachnoiditis); or nonspecific.

SPECIFIC

If the subarachnoid space is violated at the time of chymopapain injection, the most profound specific complication of the use of this drug, a subarachnoid hemorrhage may occur and, indeed, may kill the patient or permanently impair cauda equina neurological function.

Assuming your skills and temptations are such that you will never commit this error, we can discuss the specific procedure-related complications that are an accepted risk for the patient.

Muscle Spasm

Approximately 20% of patients have severe muscle spasm immediately following injection. It is manifested by back pain that is so severe that the patient is unable to move. The distress is totally incapacitating for its duration but rarely persists beyond 24 hours.

Its cause is unknown. Conjecture suggests that in the absence of any other meningeal symptoms or any radicular symptoms and in the presence of severe local back pain aggravated by movement, the source of the pain is probably within the disc rather than from a change in the epidural space. The authors have repeated myelography in some of these patients who have gone on to failure because of persistent sciatica and no unusual pathology, such as arachnoiditis, has been found. This further supports the contention that the cause of this muscle spasm originates from changes within the disc space and not from an inflammatory reaction in the spinal canal. The change within the disc space may be an acute inflammatory reaction or even hemorrhage such that the intradiscal joint space behaves like any other joint space acutely distended with inflammatory exudate or blood—movement causes severe pain.

It is important to give encouragement and reassurance that the spasm reaction in no way affects the ultimate outcome. Treatment is symptomatic with appropriate doses of analgesic and muscle relaxant medication. We have used intramuscular Solu-Cortef as a single administration but its effect is questionable.

Discitis

It is interesting that over 6000 injections by the authors have not resulted in a single known bacterial disc space infection. There is no question that discitis occurs as a complication, but it is felt to be a chemical reaction within the disc space that leads to a typical clinical picture of significant back pain. The back pain does not render the patient immobile, but it may persist for several weeks or even longer. X-ray of the lumbar spine shows specific changes (Fig. 12.1). The incidence is probably less than 1%, and the treatment is simply the passage of time and various degrees of rest, from complete bed rest through brace support to modified activity, until the symptoms subside. The x-ray appearance remains unchanged long-term and is of no clinical consequence. In fact, the ultimate x-ray appearance is no different from that of some patients with degenerative disc disease, gross disc space narrowing, and the phenomenon of adjacent vertebral body sclerosis (Fig. 12.2).

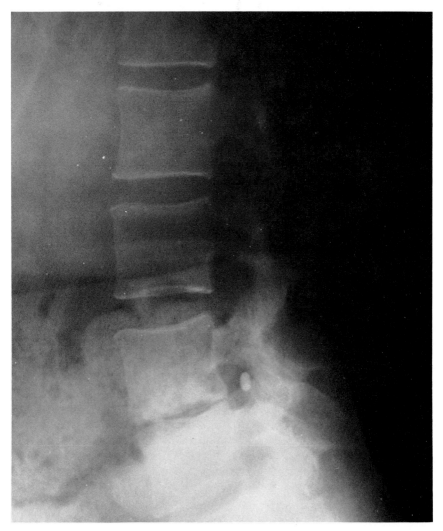

Figure 12.1.   Post-chemonucleolysis discitis at L4-5. The end plates are more irregular than in Figure 12.2.

Neurological Damage

Root Damage. The most common but still infrequent neurological complication is root damage. This occurs in one of three ways.

Under general anesthesia it is possible to penetrate the fifth lumbar nerve root on the way to the L5-S1 disc space and cause permanent damage. The authors are aware of patients in other centers who entered the hospital with S1 sciatica due to an L5-S1 herniated nucleus pulposus on one side and were discharged with a fifth root lesion on the opposite

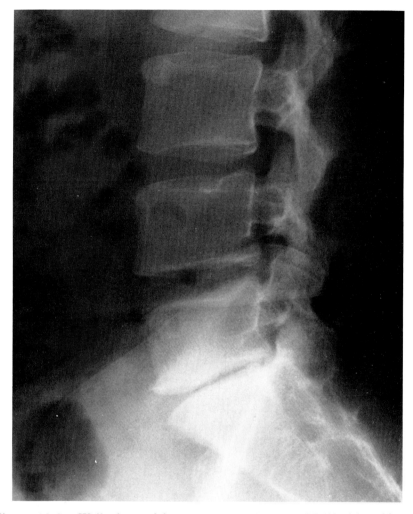

Figure 12.2. Well-advanced degenerative disc disease at L5-S1 with no history of previous disc violation by investigation or treatment. Compare with Figure 12.1.

side (side of needle entry). This neurological complication is simple to avoid. With the patient awake while the needle is advanced, it is impossible to penetrate a nerve root; the patient will simply not tolerate the pain.

The second way to impair root function is through pedicular kinking and guillotining of the nerve root. The authors do not believe this occurs for the following reasons:

a. Disc space narrowing occurs gradually in the first month and it is during this time that a neurological lesion due to kinking should become apparent.

b. We have seen no delayed increase in a neurological lesion. Everything above the disc that narrows descends: the vertebral body, the neurological structures, and the soft tissues of any nature. Thus, the pedicular descent is not isolated from the nerve root, rather it occurs in concert.

c. Bertolini and co-workers (7) have shown that progressive disc space narrowing produced slack in a nerve root rather than tension.

The third and most common reason for increased root deficit is the converison of an extruded disc to a sequestered disc by virtue of discometry too vigorously performed. The authors have two patients in whom the expulsion of a larger mass of disc material into the spinal canal has caused increased neurological damage. In both cases, the fifth lumbar root was involved; one patient was left with a significant residual weakness requiring a brace; the other patient's lesion was functionally insignificant to the patient but was readily detected on clinical examination. Although this complication is rare, gentle discometry testing is essential.

Cord and Cauda Equina Complications. Subarachnoid injection of chymopapain will result in severe cord and/or cauda equina complications, initially because of a subarachnoid hemorrhage and subsequently because of the development of arachnoiditis.

The authors have studied one known case of arachnoiditis, surgically documented and previously reported (6). The complication was felt to be due to a traumatic myelogram and the patient is still working 8 years after the event.

Preventing this complication is simple. *Do not violate the subarachnoid space at anytime during the chemonucleolysis procedure.* If you inadvertently take too vertical an approach to the disc space during needle placement and enter the foramen and subsequently the subarachnoid space, cerebrospinal fluid will flow out of the needle. The needle must be removed immediately and chemonucleolysis must be postponed for 48 hours. If an oil-soluble myelogram is used, the chemonucleolysis must not be undertaken for 24 hours, to allow the dural puncture to seal.

If myelography was very difficult, necessitating multiple punctures, wait at least 1 week before chemonucleolysis. If water-soluble myelography is used, the smaller needle required for dural puncture will allow the injection of chymopapain in a period shorter than 24 hours. An overnight wait before chymopapain injection is still recommended. If a patient has had previous back surgery with any untoward complication, such as a deep infection or a dural leak, chemonucleolysis is contraindicated. These considerations should keep you out of the subarachnoid space and avoid cord or cauda equina complications.

Retroperitoneal Hematoma

Very infrequently a patient will develop some lower abdominal crampy pain following chemonucleolysis. No actual bowel obstruction has occurred, but the reaction is thought to be due to chymopapain leaking into the retroperitoneal space and causing a small hematoma. This is only a clinical suspicion. The complication occurs so infrequently and passes without any treatment except observation. We have not witnessed this complication for some time, but now that CT scanning is available, it should be possible to demonstrate the hematoma.

NONSPECIFIC

Many adverse reactions such as myocardial infarction and thrombophlebitis are known hazards of any stressful therapeutic procedure such as chemonucleolysis, laminectomy, and discectomy. Because most patients who are admitted to the hospital for chemonucleolysis do so after a period of complete bed rest, they are at risk for thrombophlebitis. Be particularly aware of this phenomenon.

Pneumonia, cystitis, urinary tract infection, urinary retention, ileus, nausea and vomiting, headache, and meningismus are all complications that have been reported after bed rest, myelography, and chemonucleolysis. They are not considered adverse reactions directly and specifically related to chemonucleolysis.

References

1. McCulloch JA, Lorenz M: Chemonucleolysis for the adolescent patient with an HNP. To be published.
2. Hall BB, McCulloch JA: Anaphylaxis following chemonucleolysis. A review of fifteen cases. To be published.
3. Dimaio VJ: Two anaphylactic deaths after chemonucleolysis. *J Forensic Sci* 21:187, 1976.
4. Smith Laboratories, Inc. New Drug Application 18-663. Submitted to the United States Food and Drug Administration March 10, 1982 with Supplementary Data.
5. Morris J: Personal communication.
6. McCulloch JA, Canham W, Jolovich J: Chymopapain allergy: A diagnostic skin test. Submitted for publication.
7. Bertolini J, Miller J, Spencer D: The effect of intervertebral disc space narrowing on the contact force between nerve root and a simulated disc protrusion. Presented at the International Society for the Study of the Lumbar Spine Meeting, Toronto, June 1981.
8. McCulloch JA: Chemonucleolysis. *J Bone Joint Surg* 59B:45–, 1977.

Epilogue

In the field of medicine, we are being forced to examine our priorities for care, as more sophisticated techniques are prolonging life and requiring longer hospital stays. Any new concept that reduces the demand on our health care system, and at the same time offers effective, low-cost medical care will eventually prevail as the treatment of choice. Chemonucleolysis fulfills these expectations.

The second major change in our daily lives involves reexamination of the quality of life. In many parts of the world we are beyond considerations of survival and daily needs. We are seeking a full, vigorous life of purpose. We will no longer accept anything that detracts from this goal. We will not accept prolonged and unnecessary physical disability, yet at the same time we will demand the least risky, least invasive method of resolving such problems. When we look critically at simple laminectomy (discectomy) in the world literature (1, 2) and see approximately a week's stay in the hospital, a 10% complication rate, and a 10% recurrence rate, we ask if there isn't another way.

Chemonucleolysis is another effective way of managing a patient with a herniated nucleus pulposus (HNP). In our experience it has offereed a short hospital stay. The complication rate has been extremely low, and the recurrence rate even lower still.

$$\left.\begin{array}{l}\text{Least invasive}\\ \text{Least risk}\\ \text{Least cost}\end{array}\right\}\text{spinal surgery}$$

There is no question that this is an emerging trend in spinal surgery. Anyone who fails to grasp this emerging concept will be left behind by our patient population who, more and more, are insisting on this approach. Discolysis, be it with chymopapain or some other proteolytic agent, and microdiscectomy are two procedures that are least invasive, least risk, least cost. More of such procedures are sure to appear.

The struggle for clinical acceptance of chemonucleolysis has been long and hard. In 1973 and 1974, the junior author (J.M.) was ready to give up chemonucleolysis because of its variable and unpredictable results. The senior author (I.M.) offered continuing encouragement and support. He felt the problem was not with the drug but with the junior author's concept of which patient would benefit from chemonucleolysis. It was agreed that a thorough follow-up of 500 cases would be undertaken. This was a painstaking personal follow-up of patients and x-rays and computer analysis of results. The overall good results of chemonucleolysis in 43% of patients was not the least bit impressive. But the computer pointed out that patients with dominant leg pain, neurological symptoms and signs, the straight leg raising (SLR) changes described in the text, and a positive myelogram had a successful result 67% of the time. Clearly only one particular patient responded to chemonucleolysis—the patient with a clearly defined "soft" disc herniation causing sciatica and in whom a surgeon would anticipate a good result following discectomy (5).

Although the paper describing these results did not get published until 1977, the "thrill of discovery" occurred in 1975 just as the United States Food and Drug Administration (FDA) prevailed on Baxter-Travenol to withdraw their new drug application for Discase, the only commercially available chymopapain.

Many users outside the United States gave up on chymopapain. Many users continued with the drug, convinced of its efficacy, and hoped for an early solution to the controversy. Such was not to be. Battle lines were drawn and the controversy continues even as we write this epilogue. Where will it end? Hopefully the FDA's recent approval of chymopapain will reestablish the widespread and safe clinical use of chymopapain for the treatment of patients with sciatic symptoms arising from a ruptured disc.

As an aside, and of interest in the recent double blind studies, is an approximately 50% placebo response. The two major reasons for this are:
1. The placebo (saline) affected the inflammatory interface (Fig. 5.5).
2. There is a natural tendency for patients with sciatica to improve, even after "failed" conservative care.
Other considerations in evaluating the placebo response are:
1. There are much fewer excellent placebo responses than chymopapain excellent results.
2. There are more patients subsequently reclassified as failures in the placebo group.
3. Patients who would submit themselves to such a double blind study have a special kind of motivation that exposes them to placebo response.
4. Placebo response is a fact of life in any double blind study.

FDA approval is only one of the many steps chymopapain needs to regain respectability. The use of chymopapain has had two additional setbacks besides the FDA/Baxter-Travenol decision of 1975. In 1964 a patient of Brown (6) had a quadriparesis following chymopapain injection into the cervical spine. The patient subsequently died a few years later and was found to have a hemangioblastoma in the cervical cord. After the occurrence of that complication, clinical use of chymopapain was voluntarily halted briefly while its clinical use was reexamined. It was then returned to clinical use as a treatment for intervertebral disc disease of the lumbar spine.

The second time chymopapain was withdrawn from clinical use was after a report by Shealy (7) that described massive subarachnoid hemorrhage, death, and arachnoiditis in surviving cats after the administration of chymopapain. We became involved with chymopapain at this juncture, repeating Shealy's experiments but failing to duplicate his results. We concluded that chymopapain was a safe clinical tool and began our clinical use in 1969. This monograph arises out of our experiences with the drug since that time.

Thus, chymopapain is making its third comeback. Now that it is becoming available in the United States and, if users ignore the advice offered in this monograph and the experiences of many other excellent users around the world, the drug will follow a path of indiscriminate use by indiscriminate surgeons resulting in poor results and devasting complications. It would be a blow from which chymopapain will never recover. The authors hope that this scenario does not occur and that users will take time to learn more about chymopapain before administering it to a patient.

In our hands chymopapain has been a safe and effective treatment. If one reads only Chapter 12, Adverse Reactions to Chymopapain, he probably would put the monograph down and never consider chymopapain again. Perhaps we should all read Chapter 12 many times to assure that chymopapain is used safely. Then read Chapters 5 and 9 to help in the selection of patients. Then read Chapter 10 as a guide to the proper administration of the drug.

At the time of writing this monograph three commercially available chymopapain products were available: Chymodiactin, Smith Laboratories, Inc.; Discase, Travenol Laboratories, Inc., and Chemolase, Ortho-Tek, Inc. We do not feel there is any clinically significant difference in efficacy among these three products.

RESULTS

We include a section briefly summarizing our experiences that may help you inform a patient who is considering this procedure.

Many papers have been published on the results of chemonucleolysis (8–14). Most quote successful results in 60 to 80% of patients, which has been our experience with over 7000 cases.

We stress the clinical presentation of the patient and the five criteria (two symptoms, two signs, and one investigation) that constitute the diagnosis of sciatica due to an HNP (Table 7.1).

We would like to summarize our results as follows:
1. If your select patients with four or five of these criteria you can expect a good result in 70%. The rate is a little higher for the patient with an L5–S1 HNP.
2. If your select patients with mostly back pain, little in the way of leg symptoms or signs, and no supporting investigative evidence of an HNP you can expect a good result in 30% of cases which is less than placebo response.
3. When considering patients for chemonucleolysis and offering them advice for and against this treatment step we offer our experience relative to the following factors:
   a. *Age.* The average age of a patient with an HNP is approximately 40. But younger and much older patients may be seen with four or five of the clinical criteria for an HNP, and it is reasonable to conclude that they have an HNP that will respond to chemonucleolysis. Our youngest patient injected has been only 13 years old and our oldest patient 74 years old.
   b. *Sex.* We have not been able to show any better results in one sex *versus* the other. (The incidence of anaphylaxis is much higher in women.)

c. *Weight.* There does not appear to be any relationship between weight and outcome except that the very large patient is a test of your technical skills with perhaps an increased incidence of failure to place the needle in the optimum intradiscal position.

d. *Clinical Presentation.* We have not detected one particular type of presentation that separates those patients with a sequestered disc from those with other disc herniations. Except for a myelographic defect lying behind a vertebral body instead of opposite a disc space, our definition of a patient with a sequestered disc is a patient with classic sciatica due to an HNP who does not get better following chemonucleolysis.

e. *Duration of Symptoms.* It is obvious that the longer a patient is plagued by back and leg pain the more likely it is that degenerative changes will increase and the patient will develop lateral recess stenosis or spinal stenosis which will compromise root function. But you will occasionally see a patient who has had years of intermittent sciatica with relief obtained through standard conservative treatment measures, who is seen with the classic four or five criteria. You can expect a good result in this patient. However, if the patient started with the classic story of sciatica due to an HNP, but by the time you are seeing him, he has chronic backache, bilateral leg symptoms and minimal straight leg raising changes, minimal neurological symptoms or signs, and well established degenerative changes on plain x-ray, there is little hope you will help this patient by using chemonucleolysis.

f. *Disc Space Narrowing.* The degree of disc space narrowing preinjection does not influence results. Most patients, except for the very young, will have some disc space narrowing at the level of the HNP. But you will occasionally see a patient with gross disc space narrowing who still fulfills four or five of the criteria for the diagnosis of an HNP. These patients will respond to chemonucleolysis.

g. *Size of the Myelographic Defect.* We have not been able to demonstrate that a large myelographic defect is indicative of a patient who will not respond to chemonucleolysis. This is covered in more detail in Chapter 9.

h. *Previous Surgery.* If a patient has had previous successful surgery and is seen with classic sciatica due to an HNP after a latent interval of months or years, you can expect a good result to chemonucleolysis. If the recurrent disc herniation is at a different level or on the opposite side the percentage chance of a good result is no different than in the unoperated patient.

i. *Failure to Reproduce Leg Pain on Discometry (Discography).* Failure to reproduce leg pain on discometry does not mean the procedure will not be successful. Providing the patient fulfills four or five of the criteria we mention over and over, then failure to reproduce leg pain has no clinical significance (providing the position of your needle tip is perfect at the time of injection).

j. *Multiple Level Injections.* A classic disc herniation usually occurs at one level; thus, if you are injecting for the classic indication, you will be injecting single levels.

k. *Anaphylaxis.* The occurrence of anaphylaxis or other allergic reactions will not affect the outcome of chemonucleolysis.

l. *Muscle Spasm.* The occurrence of muscle spasm (20% of patients) will not affect the outcome except to prolong the patient's initial discomfort.

m. *Discitis*—The occurrence of discitis will not affect the outcome except to prolong the patient's back pain for a number of extra months. Ultimately the patient will obtain a good result.

n. *Safety.* The most striking feature of chemonucleolysis, done properly, with all necessary precautions and contraindications observed, is its safety. In our hands we have not had a serious, long-term, permanent compliation. We have not had a death.

o. *Long-Term Follow-up.* Long-term follow-up (9 years) has not demonstrated any adverse side effects locally or generally to the injection of chymopapain.

p. *Recurrence Rate.* If you obtain an initial good result to chemonucleolysis the recurrence rate at that level is very low (1%).

q. *Failure.* If the patient has disabling leg pain at 6 weeks, the procedure is considered a failure and surgery is advised. The most common cause of failure is a sequestered disc.

We feel it is appropriate to end this text with two case reports:

CASE I

D.S. is a 30-year-old lawyer from Phoenix, Arizona. She was seen with a 7-year history of back pain and a 8-month history of left sciatica unresponsive to excellent conservative care. Her leg pain was her dominant symptom. She had no neurological symptoms or signs but had a marked reduction of SLR. An outpatient CT scan supported the diagnosis of a left L4–5 HNP. She underwent an outpatient chemonucleolysis. The next day she was back home from Toronto and within 2 weeks was back to work free of leg pain. Subsequent CT scans showed a persistent defect at 1 month but at 6 months the HNP defect had disappeared (Figure 11.5).

Her sciatica was resolved without any contrast material injected into the spinal canal and without the use of an overnight hospital bed. We feel that is a remarkable achievement when compared to the standard 5- to 12-day hospital stay for myelography and laminectomy-discectomy, which are so commonly used today to handle an HNP.

CASE II

A.C. is the 43-year-old owner of a medium sized business who was seen with a 3-year history of back pain and a 4-month history of sciatica on the right side which had become his dominant symptom. His classic presentation for an S1 root lesion was diagnosed as an L5–S1 HNP on CT scan. He underwent a single level injection of chymopapain at L5–S1. He failed to improve and 2 months later underwent a microdiscectomy at L5–S1, at which time a sequestered disc was removed. The disc space was not entered at the time of surgery because chymopapain had dissolved the intradiscal nuclear material, but had failed to dissolve the the sequestered fragment which was causing continuing symptoms. Surgery was uneventful, with no adhesions interfering with exposure. The patient was discharged from the hospital the morning after surgery and returned to his office (against our advice) that afternoon. He has remained free of sciatica since microdiscectomy.

In spite of failing to respond to chemonucleolysis and requiring subsequent surgery, this man's total hospitalization was 2 days, no contrast material entered his spinal canal, and the surgical exposure of his dura and nerve root were very limited, with the assistance of the microscope, all leading to a very rapid recovery from least invasive, least risk, least cost spinal surgery.

References

1. Weir BKA, Jacobs GA: Reoperation rate following lumbar discectomy. *Spine* 5:366, 1980.
2. Shannon N, Paul EA: L4-S and L5-S, Disc protrusions: Analysis of 323 cases operated on over 12 years. *J Neurol Neurosurg Psychiatry* 42:804, 1979.
3. McCulloch JA, Ferguson JM: Outpatient chemonucleolysis. *Spine* 6:606–609, 1981.
4. Macnab I, et al.: Chemonucleolysis. *Can J Surg* 14:280, 1971.
5. McCulloch JA: Chemonucleolysis. *J Bone Joint Surg* 59:45, 1977.
6. Brown JG: The enzymatic dissolution of intervertebral disc by the use of chymopapain. *Clin Orthop* 38:193, 1965.
7. Shealy CN: Tissue reaction to chymopapain in cats. *J Neurosurgery* 26:327, 1967.
8. Bouillet R, Van de Pulte L: Treatment of lumbar sciatica with chymopapain injection in the intervertebral disc. A 7 year clinical study. *Acta Orthop Belg* 45:15, 1979.
9. Javid MJ: Treatment of herniated lumbar disc syndrome with chymopapain. *JAMA* 243:2043, 1980.
10. Parkinson D, Shields C: Treatment of protruded lumbar intervertebral discs with chymopapain. *J Neurosurg* 39:203, 1973.
11. Ravichandran G, Mulholland RC: Chymopapain chemonucleolysis; a preliminary report. *Spine* 5:380, 1980.
12. Smith L: Chemonucleolysis. *Clin Orthop* 67:72, 1969.
13. Weiner DS, MacNab I: The use of chymopapain in degenerative disc disease; a preliminary report. *Can Med Assoc J* 102:1252, 1970.
14. Wiltse LL: Chymopapain chemonucleolysis in lumbar disc disease. *JAMA* 233:1164, 1975.

Patient Preadministration and Discharge Instructions for Chymopapain Injection

You are coming into the hospital to have one or more discs in your low back injected with CHYMOPAPAIN. Chymopapain is an enzyme, extracted from the papaya plant. It dissolves only the jelly-like central portion of the disc, which may have slipped out of place to pinch a nerve and cause your sciatica (pain down your leg). It does not affect the gristle outer part of the disc, which constitutes the largest portion of the disc. Thus, "dissolving the disc" means that only a part of the disc will be removed; a greater part of the disc remains behind to continue to act as a cushion. In about 70% of patients treated with this drug, relief from sciatic leg pain occurs. (Please note that chymopapain is injected on only one occasion. The injection cannot be repeated. Chemonucleolysis is not a series of treatments.) If you do get relief, the enzyme chymopapain has successfully treated your problem and has allowed you to be better without an operation on your back. If you do not get relief, this means you still have a fragment of disc, or even a bone spur pressing on the nerve, and surgery will be necessary.

Before chymopapain is injected, you will undergo examination of your blood and regular x-rays of your back, if you have not had this investigation done. If you have not had a lumbar myelogram or CT scan, this special x-ray examination of your back will be done the day you are admitted to the hospital. During a myelogram, dye or contrast material will be placed in your back and x-rays will be taken, in order to see if the dye can show your slipped disc. The CT scan is a special computer x-ray that does not require injection of dye. It cannot be done in certain cases.

The day after your myelogram, or the day after you are admitted, you will undergo a chymopapain injection. In some patients this is done on an "outpatient" basis, which means you are not in the hospital overnight. Rather you are admitted to the minor surgery outpatient department on the morning of the procedure, and after your visit to the operating room, you spend another 3–6 hours with us and then may return to your home (if you are from out of town you may wish to return to your hotel room with your companion). The procedure is done in the operating room, and you will be awake to start. An anesthesiologist is present to give you medication before the injection, which will take some of the discomfort away. However, you will have some discomfort during the procedure, which will help me to select the correct disc to inject. The procedure is done with you on your side and I enter the *center* of the disc from the side. I usually go from the right side, whether your leg pain is on the right or left side.

Your discomfort during the procedure is usually not severe and will last only a few moments. Before injection of the chymopapain the anesthesiologist will give you additional light anesthesia to relieve any residual discomfort. The procedure of injecting chymopapain takes less than 1 hour.

After the injection, your leg pain *may* disappear very quickly. If you are going to fall into the 70% group of patients who end up with a good result, you will note relief of leg pain before a period of 4–6 weeks. If at the end of 6 weeks you have the same amount of leg pain that you had prior to the injection, your result will be classified as unsuccessful and will fall into the 30% group of patients who do not respond to chymopapain. This is when you need to consider an operation.

You probably will have increased back pain for 1 or 2 days after the injection. Some patients (20%) notice significant back pain, known as back spasms, immediately postinjection. The nurse will give you medication for pain upon your request. You leave the hospital 1 day after the injection, or the day of the injection if you are an outpatient. You are then left with a backache which generally subsides over a period of 1–3 months. Most of your back discomfort will be gone by 1–3 months.

Most patients like the support of a Camp corset to assist them in getting about in the first 4–6 weeks after the injection. If you already have a back brace, bring it with you to the hospital. If you do not have one, it will be ordered for you prior to your discharge at a cost of approximately $90. You are allowed as much walking activity with the support of the corset as your back pain allows.

Attached are instructions on how to look after yourself on leaving the hospital. After the enzyme is injected into your disc space and the jelly-like portion of the disc is dissolved, scar tissue forms in the disc space. It is important that you follow the discharge instructions, so that good, strong scar tissue can develop in your disc space and prevent lingering backache.

NOTE: ALLERGIC REACTIONS

Less than 1% of patients will have an allergic reaction at the time of injection of chymopapain. The reaction is known as anaphylaxis or shock. This is an easy problem to treat. Thus, on admission inform the nurse and doctors of any allergic reactions that you may have had to food, drugs, etc.

Approximately 2% of patients have a delayed (5–12 day) reaction of skin rash or hives. This readily disappears within a few days treatment with antihistamines that you may obtain from your family doctor. Neither of these reactions will interfere with your obtaining a good result to the injection.

GENERAL RULE

Once the procedure has been done your *back* discomfort is your activity guide. Activity (walking) will help your back discomfort. If you notice an increase in back discomfort or any significant leg pain with increased activity—rest.

On discharge from the hospital, your activities should be restricted in the following manner.

First Week

Remove your dry dressing in 48 hours. Get up late. Rest in the afternoon. Go to bed early. You may be driven in a car, but do not drive yourself. Do not do any heavy lifting. You may walk up stairs. You may take a shower or tub bath. Do not exercise.

Second Week

Same as for the first week, except:

You may drive your car for short distances (do not drive while under the influence of medication). You may increase activities such as sitting, standing, walking, all within limits set by fatigue. Do not exercise except for gentle swimming.

Third Week to Sixth Week

You may start light work which does not involve repetitive bending, rotation under stress, or lifting.

MEN: Office work only.

WOMEN: Office work or light housework.

Sixth Week

Start a flexion exercise program, under physiotherapy supervision. (Exercise instructions will be given when you return for a follow-up visit to the doctor's office 1 month postinjection). See my suggestion for exercises below.

Eighth Week

You may start heavier work, providing that it does not require repetitive bending, rotation under stress, lifting of more than 50 lb, or holding more than 20 lb at arm's length.

Twelfth Week

Men may return to heavy labor, avoiding abnormal stress to the back, such as heavy lifting from floor level.

DIET

I do not feel there is any special diet or vitamins that will speed up or slow down your recovery.

BRACE INSTRUCTIONS

The brace should be worn when you are up for any length of time. You do not have to sleep in your brace. It is not necessary to wear it when getting up to go to the bathroom at night. The brace will be needed for approximately 1–3 months. When you feel the brace is not helping your back discomfort, start leaving it off.

ACTIVITY LEVEL

General activities are as outlined above, but always exclude any activity that causes increased back or leg pain. By 3 months, most patients are capable of all routine activities and by 6 months, patients are capable of full sporting activities (within certain obvious limitations such as weight-lifting).

It is quite common to get occasional twinges of pain in one or both legs and it is also common to have cramps in the calf. These sensations are not of significance and will disappear spontaneously. The basic rule is: "Don't do anything that increases back *pain* or brings on leg pain." This applies to all activities including personal relationships. Do not be concerned about numbness—it is often the last symptom to disappear (weeks or even months).

When activities are increased you are bound to get some *aching* in the back as the tissues are stretched. This need not cause alarm and need not indicate any curtailment of activities.

You will note, in the beginning, that you are best resting in bed, second best up walking, third best standing, and last on your list of comfortable activities is sitting. You obviously have to sit for some things but avoid it as much as you can in the beginning. I am often asked about sleeping surfaces—sleep on whatever is comfortable in whatever position is comfortable (regular bed, hard bed, water bed, etc.).

FOLLOW-UP

If you live close by, I like to see you 1 month postinjection. At this time I take an x-ray and look for narrowing of the disc space which is a sign that the chymopapain has had an effect.

If you live far away (an airplane ride, rather than a car ride), it is sometimes more convenient for you to be seen by a surgeon in your community. A written report of the procedure and your postoperative course will be sent to your family physician or surgeon, and I would appreciate receiving a follow-up report on your progress from your physician.

LONG-TERM

I have been doing the chemonucleolysis procedure since 1969 and I do not feel there are any long-term side effects.

PAIN-RELIEVING, POSTURE-IMPROVING FLEXION EXERCISES

NOTE: All exercises are to be carried to your "point of pain" or a wee bit past. Do not over-irritate or muscle spasm will increase. If you are persistent in doing these exercises, the "point of pain" will change and normal range of motion will be obtained. These exercises should be performed not less than once daily.

POSITION: Lie on floor or other hard surface, facing upward.

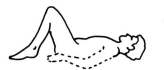 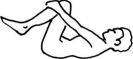 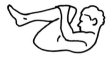

1. Draw knees up, letting feet rest flat on floor—as in position 1. Draw knees toward chest; hug knees with arms; bring head to knees. Hold 5–30 seconds. Repeat 5 times if held 30 seconds, 10 times if held less than 30 seconds.

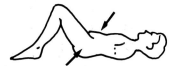 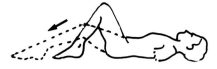

2. "Pelvic-roll or Pelvic tilt." Bend knees, letting feet rest flat on floor. Press small of back to floor by rolling pelvis forward. (To do this, tighten the abdominal muscles and pinch the buttock muscles together.) Hold this pelvic tilt and slide heels down, straightening out the legs. Rest. Then bend knees again. Rest. Then repeat 10 times.

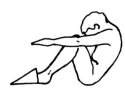 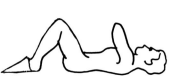 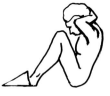

3. Sit-ups.—Bend knees. Anchor feet. Do sit-ups, curling back and keeping chin tucked toward chest. Hold arms in following manner:
   A. With arms outstretched, sit up, letting hand and forearms pass over top of knees and forehead bent toward knees. 3 times. (If you cannot do part B, do part A 10 times.
   B. With arms folded across chest and hands on opposite shoulders, sit up (curving back) and letting forehead come toward knees. 3 times. (If you cannot do part C, do part A 5 times and part B 5 times.)
   C. With finger-tips at nape of neck, come to a sitting position curving the back and letting forehead come toward knees. 4 times.

Index

Page numbers in *italics* denote figures; those followed by "t" denote tables.

Acting behavior, in exaggeration reaction
distraction testing, 89, *89–91*
specific examples, 89
Anaphylaxis, 198–202
basic science considerations, 198
classic reaction, 200
clinical considerations, 199–200
allergic history and, 200
early warning symptoms, 200
local anesthesia and, 199
incidence in chemonucleolysis, 199
management of, 200–201
antihistamines, 201
cortisone, 201
epinephrine, 200–201
IV fluids, 201
symptoms, 198–199
Angioneurotic edema, in chemonucleolysis, 202
Annular bulge
diffuse, 27, 29
disc protrusion and 29–30
localized, 29
Annulus, needle insertion and, 156, *157–158*, 159
Annulus fibrosus
biochemical makeup of, 15–16
structure and function of, 1–3, *3–5*
Anticipatory behavior, in exaggeration reaction, 91, *92–93*
Approach angle, in chemonucleolysis, 152, *156–158*, 156, 159–162, *160*, *161*
anteroposterior projection and, 152, *152–155*
higher lumbar disc spaces, 161–162
L4–5 disc space, 152, 156, *156–158*, 159
L5–S1 disc space, 159–161, *161*
lateral projection and, 151, *151*
technical considerations, 152, *153–155*

Back pain (*see also* Spinal pain)
immediately following chemonucleolysis, 182–183
intermediate postinjection course, 183–184
long-term postinjection course, 185
Bending, disc rupture and, 21

Bony root entrapment syndrome, 36–40, *37–40*
as distinguished from disc rupture
age incidence, 41
claudication, 41
multiple root involvement, 42
characteristic changes
complete cut-off of dye flow, 45, *48*
discrete myelographic defect, 45, *46*
interlaminar space narrowing, *44*, 45
subluxation, *41–43*, 43, 45
waisting of intrathecal column, *27*, 45
watershed effect, 45, *47*
chemonucleolysis and, 46, 52
claudication and, 39–42
etiology of, 36
foraminal encroachment, 36, *37*, *38*
herniated nucleus pulposus and, 39–47
midline compression, 37–39, *38–40*
myelogram limitations, 45–46
pedicular kinking, 36, *37*, *38*
subarticular, 36, *37*
Bowstring sign, 59–61, *61*
implementation, 59–60
positive, 60–61
Bursting fracture, 6

Chemonucleolysis (*see also* Lateral approach)
advantages over surgical intervention, 125, 208
basic considerations, 128
bony root entrapment and, 46, 52
case reports, 212–213
conservative care and, 121–122
contraindications, 117–118, 122–123, 197
CT scan follow-up, 191–193, *191–194*
discometry in, 167–168, 174–179, *174–177*
failure of, 186–187
general versus local anesthesia, 129–130
immediate postinjection course, 182–183
back pain, 182–183
leg pain, 183
miscellaneous observations, 183
intermediate postinjection course, 183–185
back pain, 183–184

Chemonucleolysis, intermediate postinjection course,—*continued*
    leg pain, 184
    miscellaneous observations, 184–185
    lateral recess stenosis and, 188–189
    long-term postinjection course, 185
    long-term recurrence of symptoms, 194
    multiple injection levels, *126*, 126–127
    outpatient setting, 128–129
  patient instructions, 214–218
    activity level, 217
    allergic reactions, 215
    follow-up, 217
    postinjection, 215
    procedure, 214–215
    recommended exercises, 217–218
    use of brace, 216
    week by week, 216
  patient selection, 103
    age factor, 119–120
    classic presentation, 103–106
    duration of symptoms, 120
    lateral disc herniation, 106–110, 116
    midline disc herniation, 110–113, *117*
    neurological changes, 116–119, 120t
    nonorganic factors, 121
    postsurgery, 115–116, *119*
    role of CT scan, 106, *107–115*
    spinal stenosis, 113–115, *118*
  published results, 210–212
  radiographic assessment, 186, *187*
  segmental instability and, 25–26
  situations not contraindicative
    discographic test material leak, 123–124, *124*
    sequestered disc, 123
    significant root neurological lesion, 124–125
  struggle for clinical acceptance, 208–209
  surgery following, 189–191
  technique of, 127–180
    lateral approach, 130–180
    local anesthetic routine, 130
    operating room set-up, 130–131, *131*, *132*
    tray set-up, 128, *129*
  time before relief, 185–186
Chymopapain
  action of
    in vitro, 97–98
    in vivo, 98
    instant binding, 185
    sequestered disc and, 97–98
  activation of, 99–100
  adverse reactions to, 196–207
    anaphylaxis, 198–201
    angioneurotic edema, 202
    cord and cauda equina complications, 206–207
    discitis, 203, *204*
    muscle spasm, 203
    nonspecific, 207
    preinjection testing, 202
    retroperitoneal hematoma, 206–207
    root damage, 204–206
    skin rash and itching, 202
  chemistry and tissue reaction, 97–101
  commercially available products, 210
  contraindications, 197
  handling precautions, 100
  injection of, 179–180, 196–197
  preparation of, 179
  reason for selection, 97
  reconstitution of disc, 100–101
  sequence of events following injection, 100
  toxicity of
    contrary evidence, 98–99
    form of administration, 98
    nerve fiber effect, 99
    subarachnoid hemorrhaging, 98–99
Classic presentation, for chemonucleolysis, 103–106
  dominating complaints, 103, 104, 105
  exceptions, 105
  positive ancillary investigations, 104, 105
  Rule of 5, 104–105
  signs, 103–104, 105
Claudication
  as distinguishing apophysial compression from disc rupture, 41–42
  due to bony root entrapment, 40–43
  neurogenic versus vascular, 40–41
Compression, disc rupture and, 18–19
Concealed disc, history of term, 27
Congenital lumbosacral anomaly
  disc space selection and, 138, 141–142, *141–148*, 145
  preferred terminology, 141–142, 145
Conservative care, response parameters
  degree of discomfort, 121
  degree of neurological involvement, 121–122
  degree of straight leg raising reduction, 121
  duration of symptoms, 121
  recurrence of symptoms, 122
Corporo-transverse ligament, 46–47, *52*
CT scan
  calcified herniated nucleus pulposus, *115*
  following chemonucleolysis, 191–193, *191–194*
    factors in sciatica, 193
    persistent myelographic defect, 191–193, *191–194*
  in diagnosis of herniated nucleus pulpo-

sus, 106, *107–115*
  higher thoracolumbar levels and, 106, *110–113*
  negative water-soluble myelogram and, 106, *107–109*
  sequestered disc and, 106, *114–115*
lateral disc herniation and, 106–107, *116*
lumbar root compression and, 78–79, *79*
neurological changes and, 117
showing herniated nucleus pulposus, *115–118*

Disappearing pulse syndrome, vascular claudication and, 41
Disc extrusion, 29, *30*
  association with sequestration, 29–30
  at operation, 29
Disc herniation (*see* Disc rupture)
Disc protrusion, 29, *30*
Disc rupture (*see also* specific type), 28–31
  as distinguished from apophysial compression
    age incidence, 41
    claudication, 42
    single root involvement, 42
  asymptomatic, 31
  bending and, 21
  clinical syndrome of lumbar root compression and, 54–81
    considerations, 81
    CT scan, 78–79
    discography, 78
    electromyography, 73–76
    epidural venography, 70–72
    history, 54–55
    nerve root infiltration, 79–81
    physical examination, 55–68
    radiographic examination, 68–69
  compression and, 18–19
  intervertebral disc space change and, 42–43
  L4–5 and L5–S1, *29–20*, 21
  mechanism of symptom production, 31–36
    herniated nucleus and, *33*, 34, *34*
    leg symptom and, 34–36
    location of lesion, 34
  torsion and, 19–21
Disc sequestration, 29–31, *30*
  association with extrusion, 29–30
  chemonucleolysis indication, 123
  failure of chemonucleolysis and, 186
  fragment
    location, 29
    nature, 31
    size, 30–31
  surgical correction, 189

Disc space selection, in chemonucleolysis, 136–138, *137–148*, 141–142, 145
  congenital lumbosacral anomalies, 138, 141–142, *141–148*, 145
  wrong level herniation, 135–136, 137, *137–140*
Discectomy segmental instability and, 25–26
Discitis, following chemonucleolysis, 186, *187*, 203, *204–205*
Discography
  in chemonucleolysis
    pattern of contrast material, 174–175, *174–177*
    usefulness of, 174–175
  lumbar root compression and, 78
Discometry, in chemonucleolysis (*see also* Discography), 167–168, *174–177*, 174–179
  at two levels, 178
  interpretation of, *174–175*, 178–179
  resistance to injection, 175–178, *177*
  response to injection, 178
  usefulness of, 174–175, 179
  volume of injected test material, 175–178
Distraction testing, in exaggeration reaction, 89, *89–91*
Double disc herniation, *126*
Dynasty of disc, history of 26–28

Electromyography
  lumbar root compression and, 73–76, *78*
    Hoffmann reflex, 76
    localization of involvement, 75–76
    previous spinal surgery, and 75
  normal muscle, 73
End plate fracture, 18
Epidural venography, lumbar root compression and, 70–72, *76–77*
Epiphysial ring, structure and function of, 1, *2*
Exaggeration reaction
  clinical description, 88–89, 89t, *90*, 91, *91–93*, 93–94
    acting behavior, 89, *89*, 91
    anticipatory behavior, 91, *92–93*
    characteristics, 88
    contradictory behavior, 93–94
  pentothal pain study and, 94
  psychometric testing and, 94–95

FDA/Baxter-Travenol decision, 209
Femoral nerve stretch, 64, *64*
Fogarty catheter, insertion following laminectomy, 32
Foraminal encroachment, of nerve root, 36, *37*, *38*

Herniated nucleus pulposus
  action of chymopapain on, 100
  aging and, 16–17
  anatomical location of pressure, 34
  biological basis of, 15–17
  biomechanical concepts in
    bending, 21
    compression, 18–19
    torsion, 19–21
  common neurological changes, 65, *65*
  CT scan, *115–118*
  epidemiological aspects of, 12–14
  factors affecting incidence of, 12–14
  following chemonucleolysis, 194
  in bony encroachment, 39–47
  laminectomy and, 32
  leg symptom of, 34–36
  metabolism and, 16–17
  nature of
    distension within mass, 32, *34*
    inflammation between mass and nerve
      root, 32, *34*
    mass, 32, *34*
  nutrition and, 16–17
  patient description, 31–32
  persistence of CT defect, 31, *33*
  persistence of positive myelogram, 31
  reconstitution of disc following chemo-
    nucleolysis, 100–101
  resultant nervous tissue pathology, 34
  through chemonucleolysis course, *192–
    194*
  variable effects, 35
History taking, lumbar root compression
    and, 54–55
Hoffman reflex, lumbar root compression
    and, 76
Hyaline cartilage plate, structure and func-
    tion of, 2–3, *2–3*

Instructions to patient (*see* Patient instruc-
    tions)
Intervertebral disc
  biochemical makeup of, 15–16
  extruded, 29, *30*
  intradiscal rupture, 31
  protruded, 29, *30*
  sequestrated, 29–31, *30*
  structure and function of, 1–6, *2–5*
Intradiscal rupture, as theoretical concept,
    31
Intradural tumor meniscus, myelogram, *50*

L4–5 disc space
  approach angle in chemonucleolysis, 152,
    156, *156–158*, 159
    annulus and, 156, *157–158*
    needle advancement, 159, *160*
    obstruction and, 159
    pelvic rotation and, 159
  discrete myelographic defect, *46*
  needle positioning in, *166–172*
  through chemonucleolysis course, *101*
L5–S1 disc space
  approach angle in chemonucleolysis, 159–
    161, *161*
    needle positioning and, 159–161, *161*
    obstruction and, 159–160
    unilateral sacralization and, 160
  needle positioning in, *161, 164, 166–167,
    170–172*
  through chemonucleolysis course, *101*
Lateral approach of chemonucleolysis, 131–
    180
  chymopapain injection and, 196
  phases, 131
    angle of approach, 152, 156, *156–158*,
      159–162, *160–161*
    discometric procedure, 167–168, *174–
      177*, 174–178
    injection of chymopapain, 179–180
    maintenance of proper positioning,
      132–133, *134–136*, 136
    needle insertion site, 151–152, *151–155*
    postinjection procedure, 180
    preparation of chymopapain, 179
    proper approach angle, 152, 156, *156–
      158*, 159
    proper needle position in disc, 165–166,
      166–173
    selection of correct disc space, 136–138,
      137–150, 141–142, 145
  radiation exposure and, 166
  reproduction of leg pain, 165–166, *172–
    173*
Lateral disc herniation, 106–110, *116*
  clinical presentation, 107–109
    neurological lesion, 108–110
    straight leg raising, 107, 109
  CT scan and, 106–107, *116*
  location of lesion, 106
Lateral recess stenosis
  CT scan, *51*
  disc space narrowing following chemonu-
    cleolysis and, 188–189
  failure of chemonucleolysis and, 186
  surgical correction, 189–190
Leg symptom
  areas of involvement, 34–35
  dramatic increase following chemonucle-
    olysis, 190–191
  immediately following chemonucleolysis,
    183
  in midline disc herniation, 111
  intermediate postinjection course, 184

long-term postinjection course, 185
reproduction before entering disc space,
    165–166, *172–173*
reproduction during discometry, 178
Litigation reaction
  clinical discription, 87–88
  defined, 84
Lumbar root, gross anatomical features of,
    6–7, *8*
Lumbar root compression
  anatomical variants and, 7
  clinical syndrome due to disc rupture, 54–
    81
    considerations, 81
    CT scan, 78–79
    discography, 78
    electromyography, 73–76
    epidural venography, 70–72
    history, 54–55
    nerve root infiltration, 79–81
    physical examination, 55–68
    radiographic examination, 68–69
  pathological changes and, 7
Lumbar vertebrae, gross anatomical fea-
    tures of, 1–11, *2–10*
Lumbosacral anomaly, congenital (*see* Con-
    genital lumbosacral anomaly)

Midline compression, 37–39, *39, 40*
  arthritic posterior joint overgrowth and,
    38, *39*
  as sequel to disc degeneration, 38–39
  combination of laminar and apophysial,
    38, 39, *40*
  postfusion spinal stenosis and, 38–39
Midline disc herniation, 110–113, *117*
  clinical presentation, 110–112
  population, 110
Motor loss, with root conduction impair-
    ment, 65–67, *66*
  power of ankle dorsiflexion, *66*, 66–67
  quadriceps weakness, 67, *67*
  rising on tiptoe, 65–66
Muscle spasm, in chemonucleolysis, 203
Muscle wasting, with root conduction im-
    pairment, 65
Myelogram
  bony root entrapment and, 45–46
  complete block on, *48–49*
  degenerative segmental stenosis, 25, *27–
    28*
  lumbar root compression and, 68–69, *70–
    75*
    false negative, 69
    false positive, 69
    hazards of, 68–69
    history of, 68
    procedure, 69

purposes of, 68
metrizamide, 69, *70–71, 74–75*
negative water-soluble, 106, *107–109*
oil-soluble, 69
subarticular narrowing, *51*

Needle insertion
  annulus and, 156, *157–158*, 159, *160*
  changing the angle, 155, *161–162*, 162,
    164, 165
  for single disc space injection, 162
  position in disc, 165–166, *166–173*, 196–
    197
  site of, 151–152, *152–155*
  subarachnoid space and, 196, 206
  use of bevel, 162, *163*
Nerve root (*see* Lumbar root)
Nerve root infiltration, lumbar root com-
    pression and, 79–81
  marcaine injection, 80
  needle placement, 79–80, *80*
Neurological lesion, 116–119, 120t, 124–125,
    197
  due to chemonucleolysis
    cord and cauda equina complications,
      206
    root damage, 204–206
  due to herniated nucleus pulposus, 65t
  preferred treatment, 120t
Nonorganic reaction (*see also* specific type),
    82–95
Nucleus pulposus (*see also* Herniated nu-
    cleus pulposus)
  biochemical makeup of, 16
  structure and function of, 3–4, *5*
  turgor of, 3

Oil column, waisting of, 25, *27*

Pain, assessment of, 82–95
Pathognomonic meniscus, *49*
Patient instructions, 214–218
  allergic reactions, 215
  post-injection, 215
  procedure, 214–215
  recommended exercises, 217–218
    knee hug, 218
    pelvic roll, 218
    point of pain and, 217
    sit-ups, 218
  use of brace, 216
  week by week, 216
Pedicular kinking, of nerve root, 36, *37, 38*
Pentothal pain study, exaggeration reaction
    and, 94
Physical examination, lumbar root com-
    pression and, 55–68

Physical examination, lumbar root compression and—*continued*
  bowstring sign, 59–61, *61*
  buttock tenderness, 62–63
  degree of flexion, 55–56, *57*
  extension, 55
  femoral nerve stretch, 64, *64*
  posture, 55, *56*
  root conduction impairment, 64–68
  straight leg raising test, *58*, 58–59
  tenderness and muscle spasm, 56–57
  tension and irritation, 58–64
  tests of psychogenic pain, 61–62, *62, 63*
Positioning, in chemonucleolysis, 132–133, *134–136*, 136
Positive flip test, 61, *62*
Post-chemonucleolysis course, 182–195
Prolapsed disc, lack of clinical sign for, 28
Psychogenic modification of spinal pain
  clinical description, 86–87
  defined, 84
Psychogenic spinal pain
  clinical description, 86
  defined, 83–84
Psychometric testing, in classification of spinal pain, 94–95
Psychosomatic spinal pain
  clinical description, 85–86
  defined, 83

Radiographic examination
  assessment of chemonucleolysis, 186, *187*
  lumbar root compression and, 68–69, *70–75*
Referred pain
  determinants of, 24
  hypertonic saline injection and, 24, *26*
Reflex activity, changes in with herniated nucleus pulposus, 65, *65*
Retroperitoneal hematoma, due to chemonucleolysis, 205–206
Root conduction, impairment of
  motor loss, 65–67, *66*
  muscle wasting, 65
  reflex activity, 64–65, *65*
  sensory loss, 67–68
Root tension
  bowstring sign, 59–61, *61*
  straight leg raising test, *58*, 58–59
Ruptured disc (see also Disc rupture), history of term, 27

Sacroiliac joint, 9, *10*
Sacrum, in disc space selection, 145, *149, 150*
Schmorl's node, 3, 18–19
Sciatica

associated symptoms, 24
  pathogenesis of, 24–52
  recurrence following chemonucleolysis, 194
  sources of, 24
Segmental instability, 24–29
  bilateral active straight leg raising and, 24
  diffuse annular bulge and, 25–26
  locked back and, 24
  myelogram, 25, *27–28*
  neurological examination, 25
  passive straight leg raising and, 24
Sensory loss, with root conduction impairment, 67–68
Situational spinal pain
  clinical description
    exaggeration reaction, 88–89, 89t, *90, 91, 91–93*, 93–94
    litigation reaction, 87–88
  defined, 84
Skin rash, in chemonucleolysis, 202
Spinal canal configuration, *9*
  clinical significance of, 7
  variations in, 7
Spinal fusion, segmental instability and, 25–26
Spinal pain
  classification, 82–85, 83t
    exaggeration reaction, 84
    forms of gainful alteration of health, 84–85
    litigation reaction, 84
    psychogenic, 83–84
    psychogenic modification, 84
    psychosomatic, 83
    situational, 84
  clinical description, 85–94
    psychogenic, 86
    psychogenic modification, 86–87
    psychosomatic, 85–86
    situational, 87–94
  pentothal study and, 94
  use of psychometric testing, 94–95
Spinal stenosis (*see also* Bony root entrapment syndrome), *27, 39, 40*, 113–115, *118*
Straight leg raising
  as conservative care response parameter, 121
  bilateral active, 24
  diagnostic indications, 59
  false negative, 59
  false positive, 59, *60*
  implementation, 58
  in lateral disc herniation, 107, 109
  in midline disc herniation, 111
  location of pain, 59

neurogenic claudication and, 42
passive, 24
signs of herniated nucleus pulposus, 103–
    104
tests to verify reduction, 61–62
Subarticular entrapment, of nerve root, 36,
    37, 40
Subluxation, in bony root entrapment, *41–
    43*, 43, 45

Surgery, following chemonucleolysis, 189–
    191

Torsion, disc rupture and, 19–21

Watershed effect, *47*

Zygapophysial joints, structure and function
    of, 6, *7*